Bulletproof

THE COOKBOOK

125 RECIPES TO KICK ASS

Lose up to a Pound a Day,
Increase Your Energy,
and End Food Cravings for Good

Bulletproof

THE COOKBOOK

DAVE ASPREY,
author of the *New York Times*
bestseller *The Bulletproof Diet*

RODALE

RODALE wellness

Live happy. Be healthy. Get inspired.

Sign up today to get exclusive access to our authors, exclusive bonuses, and the most authoritative, useful, and cutting edge information on health, wellness, fitness, and living your life to the fullest.

Visit us online at RodaleWellness.com
Join us at RodaleWellness.com/Join

Rodale books may be purchased for business or promotional use or for special sales. For information, please write to: Special Markets Department, Rodale Inc., 733 Third Avenue, New York, NY 10017.

Printed in the United States of America
Rodale Inc. makes every effort to use acid-free ♾, recycled paper ♻.

Book design by Amy C. King
Photographs by Mitch Mandel
Food styling by Paul Grimes
Prop styling by Stephanie Hanes

Library of Congress Cataloging-in-Publication Data is on file with the publisher.

ISBN-13: 978-1-62336-603-2

Distributed to the trade by Macmillan
2 4 6 8 10 9 7 5 3 1 hardcover

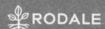

We inspire and enable people to improve their lives and the world around them.
rodalebooks.com

To my wife, Dr. Lana, who tirelessly supports my crazy biohacking
in the kitchen . . . and everywhere else.
Thank you, Lana!

CONTENTS

INTRODUCTION

IF SUPERMAN SWEARS BY IT . . . .

The best way to learn about the benefits of becoming Bulletproof is to hear from someone who's had an amazing, transformative experience. Who more fitting than the actor Brandon Routh, who played Superman in *Superman Returns* and superhero the Atom on the hit TV show *Arrow?* He's an excellent model of Bulletproof living in a demanding, performance-based profession that requires peak physical and mental shape. Brandon is playing a superhero, and in a metaphorical sense, that's what biohacking is all about—achieving your own superstrength, and discovering abilities you didn't even know you had. Brandon is a great example of Bulletproof living because he's really felt the whole 360-degree change in every aspect of his life, from losing weight to improving brain function to better sleep and more meaningful social moments. Brandon discovered the Bulletproof approach right at a time when he was ready for an overall overhaul. He didn't really realize it at the time, but once he started experimenting, he was a fast convert and remains today one of our greatest champions.

Like any job, acting has heavy demands, but there are a whole host of factors that come into play with this particular profession. It takes a really high level of performance to be an actor. There's always a lot of pressure on set, along with marathon filming days, hot lights, intense personalities. When it's time to do your thing, you have to perform, literally and figuratively. You need stamina, energy, and all your mental capacity. You can't afford to feel weak—mentally or physically. Brandon's story can give you a picture of what it feels like to be Bulletproof in all the myriad ways he experienced his own transformation. Here's the story as Brandon told it when he visited as a guest on my podcast last year. It went something like this:

I got turned onto the Bulletproof Diet by my friend Adam Karell at a bachelor party of all places. He asked if I had heard about this approach of putting butter and coconut oil in coffee. I was skeptical but intrigued by what the blog post said about the benefits of good saturated fats. After reading more of Dave's blog posts and listening to a few podcasts, I was swayed. Two days later, I tried Bulletproof and I have not stopped since. It transformed my diet and my outlook on health, and it turned the light on in my brain that I didn't know was turned off. That's something that's hard to explain to someone who's not tried it, but it really woke up my mind. It changed my energy, my clarity in communicating with people, my sleep patterns—it just changed everything. Six months after starting Bulletproof, I landed a new Superhero role as Ray Palmer aka the Atom. Ray Palmer was to be a character full of fast-talking energy, quick wit, and charisma. My Bulletproof diet helped me cultivate the mental energy and freedom needed to play him convincingly. Plus, I needed to be in great shape for the physical demands of the job, as well as for the visual demands—the dreaded shirtless scenes!

Prior to that, I had been experimenting with veganism because the food is so good, so pure, so clean. But you could only get it in vegan restaurants or by prepping it yourself. Most omnivore places aren't prepping produce that way. So I go to this party and I learn about Bulletproof eating, and I realize that there is another option for getting powerful, pure foods that would help me perform to my potential. Suddenly everything just came together. Another lucky coincidence is that, around that time, my wife and I were having conversations about how we wanted to approach nutrition with our nearly one-year-old son after a year of breastfeeding. Going Bulletproof helped us make the decision to introduce high-quality animal fats and proteins, and the results have been pretty astounding. He's thriving. He's very verbal and, at three years old, he has a very expansive vocabulary for his age group. We feel like his nutrition and the quality of his diet have played a big part in that.

So let's talk about all the ways becoming Bulletproof affected my life—because it really did change every aspect of my being for the better. The first thing I noticed was that it changed my cravings. Suddenly, I was steering clear of Dave's "suspect foods" and eating all this high-quality fat, and I just didn't crave sweets anymore. It really reset my body, too, so that if I didn't get enough fats, I'd start craving sweets again. With this new style of eating, I didn't need to snack, I didn't feel unsatisfied, and I really trusted my system to tell me what was what. Now I typically go seven to eight hours totally satiated and fully energized. When I used to get hungry, I'd get cranky, as many people do. Now, I don't have the hunger cravings, and I don't have the accompanying grumpiness. The first thing you'll notice about becoming Bulletproof is that it puts everything in better balance.

I also quickly noticed a dramatic change in my energy. It's shifted so much that it's actually changed my social demeanor. I used to be an introvert at parties; I would rather observe conversation than join in. Now, it's a total role reversal. I'm eager to engage, and my friends make fun of me because I won't shut up. I'm just bursting with energy and my mind is alert and active all the time.

And if the energy was an amazing revelation, imagine how I felt about the weight loss. I lost over 20 pounds in the first four or five months. I had been working hard and working out regularly, but it was the change in my eating that really dropped the weight. It's amazing to imagine that I starting adding high-quality fats into my diet and then watched my body fat start melting away. I also had strength gains while eating more high-quality fats and fewer carbs. As I became Bulletproof, I actually regained some youthful stamina that I assumed I had outgrown.

During this time, I also cut out drinking. I learned that, unfortunately, beer is one of the worst alcohol choices because it contains gluten and a specific mold called ochratoxin A, the same mold toxin that is commonly found in foods like coffee and chocolate. It affects the human body's performance because it causes oxidized DNA *damage, disrupting cell membranes and inhibiting the optimal functioning of mito-chondria. For this reason, beer is one of the worst alcohol choices.*

Up to this point, beer had been my drink of choice. But once I cut it out, I started feeling so much energy, I didn't even want it anymore. Now that I've cut out gluten, I can feel the toll it takes on my body—migraine headaches, bloating, brain fog, and low energy for days after consuming it. I've come to realize it's a Kryptonite food—not doing anyone any favors. I mean, I'm not an absolutist. I will have a drink once in a while, but if I do, it's usually vodka or another distilled spirit, which are the cleanest options out there.

The next thing I noticed was my cognitive function, and in particular, my memory. As an actor, I have to memorize lines. That's my job. Before I went Bulletproof, some-times I'd have bad days, brain fog, and fatigue. But now, it just comes so easily. That brain fog is all cleared up and memorization is just no big deal.

Last, but not least, I feel like becoming Bulletproof has even transformed my subtle awareness and my sense of spirituality. These days, it's almost as if I have the concen-tration of a Zen monk. I'm more self-aware, more patient, less judgmental. I also have more meaningful internal dialogue about my feelings as they arise, and I find myself to be exceedingly calm about interacting with and appraising other people. Being Bullet-proof isn't just about the body and the mind—although you'll feel those things pro-foundly. The whole thing goes deeper than that. It has the ability to shift you at your very core.

I'd like to close with a direct quote from Brandon, from that podcast, which really under-scores the transformative nature of this work.

Pay attention to your fear. Fear stops us from doing a lot of great things. I've had to find where the fear resides in me. Even though I've been fairly successful in my career, fear creeps in, doubt, self-doubt as an actor. How you present yourself to the world, what do other people think of me? I found that fear doesn't serve me when I find it. When I have the awareness to look back, when I take responsibility and find the gratitude, sometimes I find the fear underneath there. That just helps me open up and just experi-ence more and share more and have a happier, upgraded existence.

Hearing Brandon speak about his experience with going Bulletproof just makes me feel elated. This guy is as close to a superhero as it gets. He achieves that level of performance every day—mentally and physically. Since he's an actor, he's really the perfect case study. And the fact that he credits the Bulletproof Diet with helping him be his best is just the greatest reward for me, personally.

CHAPTER 1

THE BULLETPROOF PRINCIPLES

Maybe you're reading this book and already biohacking your way to Bulletproof living. You may listen to every episode of Bulletproof Radio, read every word on the Bulletproof blog, and constantly refine your program to achieve optimal performance. You may even decide to skip straight to the recipes because you've seen the incredible results the Bulletproof approach offers, and you just can't wait to get straight to the delicious Bulletproof food. And that's OK. However, whether you're new to Bulletproof or an experienced biohacker, take the time to read this opening chapter as a reminder of why we do what we do, and a refresher for the basic principles that define being Bulletproof.

First and foremost, this is a cookbook, a collection of Bulletproof recipes designed to make eating within the plan easy and satisfying, not to mention enjoyable. But before we roll up our sleeves to get into ingredients and food preparation, I'd like to underscore the foundational ideas that informed the creation of the recipes and also answer some common questions about the Bulletproof Diet. If you're new to all things Bulletproof, this chapter will give you a solid orientation to the philosophy, research, and goals that lead to the Bulletproof state of high performance. These are lessons with the power to change your life. Becoming Bulletproof isn't a quick fix or a fad; it's a new way to understand your physical state and tweak it to bring out unforeseen levels of energy and functionality.

It's not about being invincible. It's about adding so much to your energy and willpower reserves that you feel you can "bring it" no matter what life brings your way. For me, when I weighed 300 pounds, I honestly felt I didn't have that strength or control. Now, my joy and potential feel limitless. Becoming Bulletproof is about your true resilience, and realizing that you can do anything you set out to accomplish.

So before we get into recipes, let me outline the top tenets of the approach, and boil it down to basics to help organize the most important takeaways. The following sections will give you a good 101 understanding of what it is we're doing here, and why it works. From the top, here are the most common questions I'm asked about the Bulletproof Diet.

WHAT DOES IT MEAN TO BE BULLETPROOF?

Becoming Bulletproof is, in the simplest terms, about making you the most powerful being you can be, in terms of physical performance, brain power, and all-day energy. That means getting the very best out of your body and brain, all of the time. When I started this quest, I weighed 300 pounds. And while I was a fabulously successful entrepreneur in Silicon Valley, my physical and mental state was in sad shape. Because I had a background in tech, I understood the concept of hacking in a very real way. I had personal experience encountering barriers and boundaries and learning how to decode and work around them. So I employed that same approach in trying to figure out and conquer my weight problem and foggy brain. I believed on a gut level that there were ways to decode my system and create workarounds that would give me greater control over my system—not to outsmart it, but to understand its inner workings and optimize the functionality that my body, in its best state, could deliver.

As it turned out, this approach changed my life—and the lives of hundreds of thousands of people after me. All of my methods are driven by the idea that we are constantly refining and learning about what works for us personally, and making small tweaks—just as one does in technology—to make our bodies smarter, stronger, and more robust. There is no magic bullet. But if you can reset your body to cut your cravings, you'll change the state of your body and mind.

WILL THE BULLETPROOF DIET HELP ME LOSE WEIGHT?

Yes, being Bulletproof is a way to lose weight. It transforms the body into a lean, efficient, energetic machine. But that's really only a side effect of getting your body to operate in its most efficient state. Did I want to lose weight? Hell, yes. Is that why most people try the Bulletproof Diet in the first place? Absolutely. But is that what we're really doing here? No. Becoming our best, most powerful selves means fine-tuning every system in the body, from metabolism to detoxification to brain power. And when we do that, we lose excess weight because our systems are acting as they should. They are working at max

capacity while burning energy efficiently and consistently. In essence, weight loss is a byproduct of making the body function optimally. I won't lie—it's the byproduct that most of us care the most about. But a thousand other good things are happening that make the weight loss possible. That's why becoming Bulletproof creates a noticeable upswing in brain function and energy levels. That's why people report feeling amazing—the best in their lives—when eating this way. So yes, weight loss is an awesome thing. But it's not the only thing. And it's not the thing that defines Bulletproof living. Bulletproof is much more concerned with holistic success, measured by performance across a number of bodily and brain functions.

HOW DOES THE BULLETPROOF DIET WORK?

The Bulletproof Diet doesn't work like most diets—there's no calorie counting because when you stop eating foods that make you weak, you'll actually be able to hear the hormone hunger signal from your body, and you won't experience food cravings. You don't have to attempt to magically work out more than you eat, which creates unsustainable biological stress for most people. And let's remember, famines and labor camps are not great ways to build willpower or resilience.

Instead, choose foods that have the right kind of energy, but are also lowest in the things that slow you down, and highest in nutrients. Then, you eat them at the time when they will do the most for your body and mind based on circadian biology. This is a far cry from most "healthy" diets, which focus on decreasing the amount of energy in your food while increasing the amount of nutrients and totally ignoring the effects of antinutrients.

The Bulletproof Diet partially falls into a category broadly known as ketogenic diets, though my plan has fewer ketones than a full-on ketogenic diet. (For you science geeks out there, it's a cyclical ketogenic diet with nutrient timing!)

You've probably heard of plans like the Atkins Diet and the Paleo Diet, which also fall under the ketogenic umbrella, but make no mistake: The Bulletproof Diet is different from those popular programs, for reasons I'll get to shortly. The thing that lumps these approaches into a single category is the way that weight loss is achieved, namely by a process called ketosis. Ketosis is a state wherein your body burns fat instead of carbs. When you think about it, this is a pretty simple proposition. Your body typically burns carbs, turning them into sugar for energy. But if your body is out of carbs, it will go to Plan B: fat burning. It's a natural function, and one that your body would employ in a natural

way depending on your circumstances. If you found yourself in a situation where you were deprived of carbs, your body would know what to do, and would find an alternate energy source (read: your stored fat). The Bulletproof Diet is built around creating a ketogenic state in order to burn fat stores for energy rather than using carbs. When you carb-load, you're stockpiling your body with extra energy to use, but in the absence of those carbs, your body will burn fat, so you become leaner in the process.

IS KETOSIS SAFE?

When I was initially discovering the power of ketosis for myself, I'd heard about the so-called Eskimo diet, where almost no calories come from carbohydrates, and most calories come from fat. Nutritional alarmists will often confuse a state of metabolic keto-acidosis from diabetes with the completely natural form of ketosis from diet—it's a natural state in which the body rests. Full ketosis is used to treat epilepsy and cancer, even in kids, with great safety. In this state, your body creates carbs from proteins. For some people, this is optimal and they stay in this state for prolonged periods. For other people, like me, it makes me feel run down. This is why, for ultimate resilience—and especially for women—I recommend cycling in and out of ketosis. I recommend eating some carbs as it stresses the body to create carbs from protein. With my recommendation, you get the best of both worlds. And my recommendation is still less suggestive of a ketogenic state than most paleo diets recommend.

When I began studying ketosis, I wanted to see what would happen if I entered a ketogenic state and stuck with it indefinitely—or for three months, as was the case for me. Guess what? It wasn't good. The Inuit people subsist primarily on protein and a huge amount of fat. They live on delicacies like whale blubber and seal jerky. And good for them; they are genetically predisposed to function this way as they've evolved with this diet for centuries . . . and they live on packed snow. We, in everyday America, however, have not. After eating nothing but protein and ridiculous amounts of fats for three months, my body started malfunctioning. My sleep quality went away. My eyes and sinuses were superdry all the time. I started getting headaches. Because I didn't have enough carbohydrates to manufacture the mucus that lines a healthy stomach, I developed food allergies to my favorite foods as soon as I added them back in. I'm still working to hack the food allergies I developed by eating that way, and making great progress. Clearly for me, this state of prolonged ketosis was a terrible idea. I know that having experienced it firsthand, and I've seen lesser versions of these symptoms—especially

sleep and energy problems—in a good number of Bulletproof followers who stay in ketosis for long periods, though not all of them. This is why the Bulletproof approach advocates moving in and out of a ketogenic state, always being mindful of how and when we eat carbs for added energy. For the vast majority of people, I do not advocate putting your body in a ketogenic state indefinitely.

What I do know is that you can use ketosis as a tool, in measured, regular bursts, to bring out some amazing fat-burning and brain-revving potential. That is what being Bulletproof is all about: biohacking your way to the sweet spot where your system thrives and continually outperforms itself without causing damage or detriment to your systems.

SO HOW IS THE BULLETPROOF DIET DIFFERENT FROM THE ATKINS AND PALEO PLANS?

The Bulletproof Diet recommends 6 to 11 servings of veggies a day. "Whoa" you're thinking. "That's a ridiculous amount of veggies." And you're right. Some people have a hard time adjusting to eating this many servings of veggies because it so far exceeds what we've become accustomed to in the sad state of an American diet devoid of nutrition. I'm advocating more veggies per day than most other programs, and even some vegan diets!

The FDA recommends 5 servings of ½ cup (or 2½ cups per day). But please note, they treat fruits and veggies as the same thing. This is a flawed approach, because fruit is mostly sugar, while vegetables are mostly nutrients and fiber. I recommend 9 servings of veggies a day and potentially a lot more. So my plan suggests at least three times more than the FDA recommends. That's important to remember, because while we're asking you to skip carbs, in measured cycles, we're also flooding your body with the amazing nutrients nature provides, and teaching you how to identify and limit carb-heavy, starchy vegetables, except when you want your body to have healthy carbohydrates. So that's the first way Bulletproof living is different from the Atkins plan.

Atkins and Paleo are both considered "low-carb high-fat" (LCHF) diets. Atkins focuses on a high-protein, high-fat eating plan to trigger ketosis, but doesn't focus on the type of fat or protein. Paleo also advocates a high-protein, high-fat diet, but it does pay attention to the *type* of fat and protein, which is a major improvement. But it's also high enough in protein to trigger inflammation, and the impact of cooking techniques isn't a part of the diet, even though it affects how you use your food.

The Bulletproof Diet is also an LCHF diet, like Paleo and Atkins, but it has compo-nents that set it apart entirely: namely, a focus on eliminating cravings by controlling food toxins, and eating the right foods at the right times, not to mention significant differences in Bulletproof cooking methods. People forget that cooking is a form of food processing, and you can "process" food in your own kitchen and accidentally turn it from something nutritious into something that will make you crave sugar. This should be a no-brainer, but plenty of other diets don't really take this aspect of the formula into consideration.

Other plans know that by introducing ketosis, the body will burn fat, and so they figure, mission accomplished. But if you're burning fat that's full of food toxins, you're going to experience fatigue and cravings . . . totally not Bulletproof!

The Bulletproof Diet also differs from the Atkins and Paleo diets in its attention to toxins, or antinutrients. As I was hacking my own performance, and losing 100 pounds, I learned a lot about the toxins that exist, naturally and unnaturally, in our food supply. Besides of all the manmade toxins that have entered our food chain via pesticides and manufacturing processes, there are also naturally occurring antinutrients that, while they won't kill us, can slow down or compromise our natural system functions. Take kale, for example. The darling of healthy eaters everywhere, kale is enjoying its moment in the sun. It's all the rage in salads, juices, pastas, you name it. Every hip restaurant has kale somewhere on its menu, and most markets now offer an array of heirloom varieties. Here's the thing. Kale isn't always good for all of us. It's a goitrogenic food, which means that in its raw form it interferes with iodine uptake and can cause enlargement of the thyroid (this is where the term goiter comes from). It can slow your thyroid function, which is a bad thing because your thyroid controls your energy levels.

Fortunately, most of us will never experience this side effect. You'd have to eat kale in large amounts to see this come to pass. That said, with the obsessive embrace of kale in recent years, plenty of people do drink a glass of kale juice and eat a kale salad or two every day. If you already have compromised thyroid function, this could very well lower your performance even more. More worrying, kale is high in oxalic acid, a compound that prevents most animals from eating raw kale because it increases the kidney load. Excessive oxalic acid is tied to gout and even a condition where oxalic acid crystals form in your vagina, making sex painful. This is why the Bulletproof plan is on a spectrum. I highlight certain foods that have the potential to cause nonoptimal effects, like kale. It doesn't mean it will cause serious injury, but it does mean your body has to work that much harder to process what it perceives to be a low-grade poison. This is why I recommend skipping—or specially prepping—what I call "suspect foods," acknowledging that they contain a meaningful amount of antinutrients.

Another example is quinoa. People freak out when I say to avoid quinoa! After all, it's recently been touted as nature's perfect superfood. Like kale, it's enjoying its 15 minutes. But research shows us that quinoa is coated with saponin, which is a common cause of food allergies. When we consume saponin, it can create small holes in the membrane of cells in your gut and it can irritate the immune system. The saponin is there to protect the grain from fungal infection, but when we remove the saponin (by processing and rinsing with water), the quinoa is vulnerable to mold growth, and mold makes a host of well-known toxins that make humans weak. Like all grains, quinoa is susceptible to spoilage, which is why I recommend choosing rice instead—it's the least likely to spoil.

So when I advise against incorporating quinoa, it's not because I'm some guy who thinks quinoa makes you fat or something; it's because I've flagged it as a food that can compromise your system from optimal function, so I'd prefer to find other foods that are easier for us to process and contain fewer likely antinutrients. In Bulletproof lingo, quinoa is a "suspect food"—it's not on the Kryptonite list, but it's far from a superfood. Blindly loading your plate with it won't get you the results we seek.

The third reason the Bulletproof Diet is different than other LCHF diets is that we pay attention to the way we prepare food, as that can change the chemical makeup of the ingredients. Food preparation can make food taste better. Sometimes it makes food's nutrients more absorbable. But sometimes food is cooked to the point of making it inflammatory or even carcinogenic. Excessive cooking or heat not only strips food of its nutritional value, it actually causes it to become actively harmful. This is a huge deal, so you'll notice in my recipes that I'm particular about which foods are eaten raw and which are prepared using what methods. Again, this isn't some flight of fancy; this is based on research that indicates that we can debase foods to a harmful state. And you don't have to do it perfectly . . . a little raw kale won't hurt you. But a lot is not a great idea. Knowing this helps you make better food choices, and makes you a better cook.

One of the latest culinary trends in recent years is molecular gastronomy, or modernist cuisine. This approach applies biology and science to cooking, using lab techniques to change the nature of food into surprising textures and flavors—it's precisely changing the chemical compound of foods for maximum flavor, no matter what. As with all top-tier cuisines, it's done in a dazzle-you dog-and-pony show that elicits *oohs* and *ahhs* for a big wow factor. And some of it tastes pretty amazing, too. But here's the thing: I don't care if it tastes amazing. Food that is overprocessed and engineered in a factory or in your kitchen, treated as though it's a lab element, often is so damaged by the processing that it tastes good but makes you weak. It loses its essential nature, becomes inflammatory in nature (which means you get cravings when you eat it), and adds toxins into the mix based on the processing it undergoes. The good news is, you don't have to choose between food that tastes fantastic and offers you incredible results in terms of boosted energy and optimal performance. My recipes are as flavorful as they are functional.

The Bulletproof approach is all about using a precise understanding of food chemistry so that we can prepare food that delivers maximum nutrition and minimum inflammation, and tastes great too. The Bulletproof approach is all about cooking to achieve a state of wellness for greater performance. The end result of using my recipes should be that you feel amazing, have increased energy, and enjoy an anti-inflammatory meal that tastes fantastic. Eat amazing foods, prepared the right way, and get ready to feel a real food high.

DOES THE BULLETPROOF DIET RECOMMEND FASTING?

Yes and no. If fasting means starving yourself and eating nothing for days, that's not a part of it. Instead, the Bulletproof Diet helps you avoid some types of foods at certain times so you can get the benefits of fasting without the energy crashes. The way the Bulletproof Diet works best is to adopt the recommended Bulletproof Roadmap of foods (go to www.bulletproof.com/diet-roadmap-poster to get the Bulletproof Diet Roadmap downloadable poster), use the recipes in this book, and then practice two occasional types of fasting to kick-start weight loss, reduce inflammation, detox your cells, and supercharge your results. The two types of fasting I recommend are Bulletproof Intermittent Fasting and Bulletproof Protein Fasting, both of which I detail below.

BULLETPROOF INTERMITTENT FASTING

Bulletproof Intermittent Fasting requires far less willpower than any other type of fasting. In fact, it requires none at all. This technique is popular in biohacking circles because it not only promotes fat loss, it also builds muscle, fights disease-causing

WHEN TO EAT

The Simple Bulletproof Diet

Designed to reduce body fat, enhance mental performance, and prevent disease while leaving you satisfied and energized.

Eat when you're hungry, stop when you're satiated, and try not to snack. Target 50–70% of calories from healthy fats, 20% from protein, 20% vegetables, and 5% fruit or starch. For optimal results, follow the dark portion of the diet and limit fruit or starch consumption to 1–2 servings per day in the evenings to avoid high triglycerides.

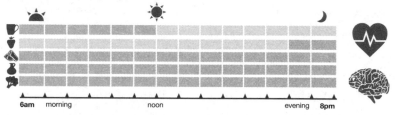

Bulletproof Intermittent Fasting for Fat Loss and Focus

A biohack that makes it possible to lose fat, while increasing mental focus and energy, without cravings.

You start by consuming a cup of Bulletproof Coffee in the morning. The healthy fats give you a stable current of energy, and the ultra low-toxin Bulletproof Coffee beans optimize brain function and fat loss. For optimal results, follow the top portion of the diet in conjunction with this protocol.

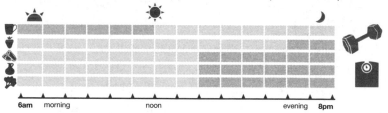

Bulletproof Protein Fasting

A biohack used occasionally to get a greater reduction in inflammation.

About 1–2 times a week, limit your protein intake to 15–25g to help cleanse your inner cells without muscle loss. To keep you full and energized, consume a cup of Bulletproof Coffee in the morning and have high fats and moderate carbs throughout the day. For optimal results, follow the top portion of the diet and limit carbohydrates to the afternoon and evening.

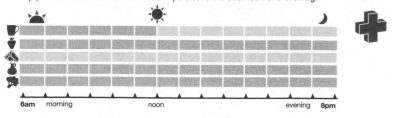

inflammation, and builds up your body's resilience by burning more fat, which helps the body produce less insulin. The main idea behind traditional intermittent fasting is that you eat all your food for the day in an 8-hour period, then fast the rest of the time. Bulletproof Intermittent Fasting, on the other hand, is a fundamentally new and different idea I originated, and it solves the problem of regular fasting. With traditional fasting, you might skip breakfast, have a late lunch at 2 p.m., and eat dinner before 8 p.m. The rest of the day you wouldn't eat, and you would likely get hungry and weak around 11 a.m. when you're working a normal job. For people who have a significant amount of weight to lose—like more than 30 pounds—fasting can be distracting and can affect mental and physical performance, which is why Bulletproof Intermittent Fasting (see a sample day on page 213) is such a great solution for getting the benefits without the negative side effects.

If you're a busy entrepreneur or a student, and you're really relying on your mental power being in top form 24/7, you will probably find with traditional intermittent fasting that you are hungry and tired at 11 a.m., which stresses your adrenals to keep your blood sugar up. By adding Bulletproof Coffee (with no protein or carbs of any kind) during your "fasting" time, you can experience a complete lack of hunger and full-power

energy while getting the benefits of an intermittent fast. The cool thing is that an all-fat breakfast (like Bulletproof Coffee) won't make your body think it's broken the fast, so you get the benefits of the fasting without feeling deprived. It's awesome!

Now let's talk a little bit about why Bulletproof Intermittent Fasting works better than traditional intermittent fasting. It's because of mTor, a major mechanism that increases protein synthesis in your muscles. Both exercise and coffee raise your energy while simultaneously inhibiting your muscle-building mechanism (that's the mTor) for a short while, causing it to "spring back" and build even more muscle as soon as you eat something.

Therefore, in order to build muscle you must suppress mTor; the muscle building happens when the mTor surges after being suppressed. So anything that helps you push it down hard means it will surge even harder, which in turn helps you gain muscle. Ways to suppress mTor include intermittent fasting, exercise, and coffee or, on a lesser scale, chocolate, green tea, turmeric, and resveratrol. So guess what? Bulletproof Intermittent Fasting can make your mTor bounce back. When I started playing around with this concept and figured out how to maximize my mTor supression, I went from 300 pounds to a lean machine with a six-pack in 18 months, despite consuming 4,000 calories a day with no exercise. Plain intermittent fasting doesn't use coffee, so it only hits one, or possibly two of the three possible mTOR suppressors. Bulletproof Intermittent Fasting works better because it can use all three mechanisms: intermittent fasting, exercise, and coffee.

The next reason Bulletproof Intermittent Fasting is superior to regular traditional intermittent fasting is because one of the ingredients in Bulletproof Coffee increases the speed at which you go into ketosis, fueling your brain and helping you maintain a ketogenic state, even in the presence of some carbs in your diet. We use XCT oil, which works because it spikes molecules called ketones in the blood the fastest and highest. Ketones are produced by the liver from fatty acids during low food intake periods. A momentary spike in these ketones suppresses hunger, so while fats like coconut oil and plain MCT oil don't spike it enough to fully feel this effect, XCT oil does the trick as it contains C8 and C10, an optimal combination of fatty acids. It creates ketones because it is metabolically unique as a fat, and some parts of the brain prefer fuel from fats to that derived from carbs.

For all these reasons, it just makes sense to add Bulletproof Coffee to the equation. It's easier, and far more pleasant to do a Bulletproof Intermittent Fast than a plain fast. I've done plain ones and enjoyed them to be honest, but they are even more enjoyable with Bulletproof Coffee. Besides, coffee increases your metabolism by up to 20 percent. So for my money, Bulletproof Intermittent Fasting—with coffee—is vastly superior in terms of satisfaction and results.

BULLETPROOF PROTEIN FASTING

Protein fasting means that one day per week, you eat almost no protein—no more than 15 grams. The reason we do this is because when the body doesn't have any protein, it induces autophagy—or, literally translated, self-digestion. Yes, that's just what it sounds like. It means your body uses the enzymes that were intended to digest protein to digest waste inside your cells instead. Our cells accumulate waste and toxic junk, which slows us down and causes aging. When we biohack our way into autophagy, we fight back, clearing away this bodily waste and giving our cells a new lease on life. Suddenly, your body feels lighter, and your brain feels brighter.

I recommend you add a protein fasting day to your regular Bulletproof eating once a week. If it makes it easier, choose the same day each week and just get into the habit of skipping protein that day. Once you get the hang of it, Bulletproof Protein Fasting just becomes another part of your routine, and one that brings great benefits when you're biohacking your system. Here's why: Protein fasting improves cellular repair function. The enzymes from your pancreas and liver, besides removing toxins, remove debris from your cells. Protein fasting improves mitochondrial function, because autophagy is the sole known mechanism for replacing mitochondria. And when your cells are functioning better, so will you. Protein fasting also upgrades your brain's ability to drain waste through the glymphatic system and promotes better sleep—another key way to improve your mental and physical performance.

You're probably asking how you're going to get energy and feel full if you're cutting out protein, but remember, you can get plenty of energy and satiety from good fats. Start your day with Bulletproof Coffee for a hit of healthy fats and caffeine, and then eat high fats and moderate carbs throughout the day. You'll find sample meal plans for protein fasting days in the appendix. For best results, limit the carbs to later in the day, which improves sleep quality. It may sound simple enough, and it will be when you get used to it, but be aware: Protein lurks in unexpected places. Broccoli? There's protein. You'll also need to be careful about serving sizes. Anything with less than 1 gram of protein can be labeled as 0 grams according to the FDA—so watch the amount of any foods that may contain protein, even in small amounts (vegetables and even coconut milk, for example), which may contain trace amounts not listed on the label.

When you commit to Bulletproofing yourself, protein fasting is one of the most powerful tools in your arsenal. It's also great because you can use it in a routine way, like once a week, or when you're feeling sluggish, or when you have compromised immunity.

BULLETPROOF PROTEIN FASTING

Bulletproof Protein Fasting is a biohack to get a greater reduction in inflammation and to kick-start weight loss. For new readers and routine followers of the Bulletproof Diet alike, it is a day of protein fasting once each week, where you eat virtually no protein: limit your protein to 15 grams or less per day. To keep you full and energized, consume a cup of protein-free Bulletproof Coffee (page 166) in the morning and have near-zero protein, high fats, and moderate carbs throughout the day. For optimal results, limit carbohydrates to the afternoon and evening.

Use this tool to give your cellular function a boost when you need it most. Autophagy is also required to maintain muscle mass, as it inhibits muscle breakdown in adults, so it has the dual benefit of making your system perform better while your body looks better.

As with any sort of dieting or fasting, going overboard will likely have adverse effects on both your body and your brain. If you become chronically protein deficient, your body will suffer. Over time, insufficient protein will cause decreased immune function, muscle mass, and bone density, as well as reduced endurance. When I first started experimenting with protein fasting, I tried reducing my intake to 25 grams per fast day. But when I pushed further, I discovered that limiting my intake to 15 grams per day really produced the miraculous results I wanted— as long as I did it in limited bursts. In no time, I reduced abdominal inflammation and lost my muffin top. (And yes, even biohacked Bulletproofers are prone to the dreaded muffin top once in a while!) Protein fasting feels like a deep clean that reinvigorates my whole body, right down to the cellular level. The trick is to biohack autophagy in short, temporary bursts for 24 hours at a time. That way, you get all the benefits without the negative side effects.

Like just about everything I advocate, Bulletproof Protein Fasting is not black and white. Everyone will have their own response to it at varying degrees of application. I recommend trying different amounts of protein to see what works best for you. That's the essence of biohacking—learning what works best for your body. I would caveat this to exclude pregnant women, for whom I don't think fasting—either intermittent or protein—is a great idea. If you're eating for two, nutrients need to be delivered steadily. You can always biohack that baby weight after a healthy birth.

SO WHAT SHOULD I BE EATING?

The Bulletproof Roadmap is your go-to guide for the best possible foods for a high-performance diet. I mention the web link below each roadmap graphic in Chapter 2 for anyone who is newly discovering the Bulletproof way of life. We'll talk more about how to approach eating and apply these principles in the coming chapters.

This roadmap is your Bulletproof bible. Take a look at the graphics, starting on page 24, to familiarize yourself with the whole ecosystem of Bulletproof eating. I've organized the foods into categories so you can easily assess which foods are optimal, and which ones are just average or potentially a poor choice. Foods from the top end of the spectrum are your best choices for your health and performance, your brain, and your body. Foods in the middle portion of the spectrum are "suspect foods." Depending on the sourcing, freshness, your own personal tolerance and food allergies, and any processing that the foods have undergone, they can be detrimental in some cases, and are probably best avoided on a regular basis.

The foods in the bottom zone are the most toxic and inflammatory, and should be avoided if at all possible. This doesn't mean that you can't ever eat the foods from this part of the spectrum. It simply means that if you decide that you want to eat those foods, you should be aware that they aren't the best foods for performance and will likely have some bad consequences, and that you should do everything you can to biohack yourself to protect your brain and body from the toxins in these foods, and to increase your resilience and ability to bounce back from the bad effects.

Getting high-quality produce and meats is essential for ensuring that you're feeding your body with good nutrients, and avoiding harmful toxins and additives. Grass-fed beef and lamb; wild-caught fish; pastured pork; and organic fruits, vegetables, and grains are all things you should be striving to eat as much as possible. People complain that these foods cost more than industrial or commercially farmed versions, but it is far cheaper to eat high-quality, toxin-free foods and to perform at a high level than it is to eat low-nutrient foods with additives and chemicals, and be spending an arm and a leg on medicine and doctor visits because you are sick all the time. If that's not convincing enough, the higher quality foods even taste better and will give you far more satisfaction when eating them!

HOW MUCH SHOULD I EAT?

There is no calorie counting or food measuring on the Bulletproof Diet. Instead, we focus on eating the right foods to supply your body with the nutrients and energy that it needs to function properly. Your body will tell you when you need more of something, and you should eat when you're hungry, and stop when you're full. The amount doesn't matter so much, however, the ratio of foods that you are eating is important.

An easy overview of your daily intake:

1. You should enjoy 5 to 9 servings of **fats** per day, making up 50 percent to 70 percent of your total calorie intake. Those fats should be of the healthy variety, like grass-fed butter and Bulletproof Brain Octane oil.
2. Your meals should be packed full of **veggies**, which are loaded with micronutrients but contain very few calories. You should have 6 to 13 servings

of veggies per day, or up to 20 percent of your total calories.

3. You should enjoy 4 to 6 servings of **protein** per day, up to 20 percent of your total calories. Eat the amount of protein that is comfortable for you. A good amount to shoot for is about 1.5 grams of protein per pound of body weight, with some starch and as much fat as you'd like.

4. I advocate eating 1 to 2 servings of **fruits and starches** per day, adding up to no more than 5 percent of your total calories. A little bit of fruit and low-toxin, starchy carbs like white rice and sweet potatoes are good to eat on a regular basis throughout the week, ideally in the evening time, but just not regularly or throughout the day.

5. And lastly, **sugars**—particularly refined sugars, sweeteners, and juices—should be avoided as much as possible.

GETTING STARTED

The principles of the Bulletproof Diet are simple; however, many people struggle with figuring out exactly where and how to start. Here is a step-by-step approach to getting Bulletproof, prioritizing the most important aspects of the diet and the things that will give you the biggest health and performance boost. Try these steps in this order and watch how quickly you start to live Bulletproof.

1. **Eliminate sugar.** This includes sweeteners like honey and agave, and also includes fruit juices and sports drinks that contain things like high-fructose corn syrup.

2. **Replace the sugar calories with healthy fats.** Get more grass-fed butter, ghee, coconut oil, and high-quality MCT oils such as Bulletproof Brain Octane oil and Upgraded XCT oil in your diet.

3. **Eliminate gluten in any shape or form.** Avoid bread, cereal, and pasta; and also don't make the mistake of switching to "gluten-free" versions of these foods, which can contain loads of other additives and be just as bad.

4. **Remove grains, grain-derived oils, and vegetable oils.** This includes corn, soy, and canola oils, as well as unstable polyunsaturated oils from walnuts, flax, and peanuts.

5. **Eliminate all synthetic additives, colorings, and flavorings.** This includes artificial sweeteners such as aspartame, additives like MSG, and any dyes and artificial flavorings.

6. **Remove all processed, homogenized, and pasteurized dairy.** If you must choose high-fat items that have been pasteurized, they should be grass-fed. Most people can tolerate full-fat, raw, whole dairy from grass-fed cows, even those with lactose intolerance.

7. **Eliminate legumes.** This includes peanuts, beans, and lentils. If you do eat beans, make sure to soak, sprout/ferment, and cook them.

8. **Eat significant amounts of wild-caught seafood and pastured, grass-fed meat.** Beef, lamb, and bison are ideal. Pastured eggs, pork, and poultry are also good meat choices.

9. **Switch to organic fruits and vegetables.** Organic is more important for some produce than others. Visit www.whatsonmyfood.org for more info.

10. **Limit fruit consumption** to 1 to 2 servings per day. Berries, citrus, and other low-fructose fruits are better choices than high-fructose fruits such as apples and watermelon

11. **Add spices and herbs.** Fresh, high-quality spices and herbs from the green side of the spectrum are the easiest ways to make your food taste delicious.

12. **Cook your food gently.** Use low temperatures and water-based cooking methods whenever possible. Avoid using the microwave and frying.

Enjoy your food. Happiness and gratitude are every bit as important as the right nutrition!

A FEW RULES OF THE ROAD

1. If you have to have some form of cheat/junk/fake food, have it, and don't act like you're "off the wagon." The more you venture from the Bulletproof Diet, the less you'll benefit. The more you stick to the Bulletproof Diet, well, the more Bulletproof you'll be. Small variations are fine and do not constitute failure.

2. If you experience allergies, acne, or other negative effects after consuming dairy, switch to ghee as your only dairy, and eat coconut oil and animal fat.

3. Eat as little polyunsaturated fat as you can. And be sure to supplement your fat intake with fish oil or krill oil if you don't consume fatty cold-water fish like salmon on a weekly basis.

4. Try not to snack. I feel confident that once you get accustomed to eating

this way, and your body fat adapts, you actually won't have snack cravings. In fact, if you follow the Bulletproof Coffee recipe with Bulletproof Brain Octane oil, you can expect to feel your cravings disappear the very first day. If you do experience cravings, turn to one of my favorite choices: cold smoked salmon and a slice of avocado. It's like the freshest, most delectable sushi, and it should immediately satisfy and give you an energy boost to sustain you until your next meal.

If you do this mostly right, you'll set yourself up for a low-inflammation, high-performance, high-energy lifestyle. If you don't make time to take care of yourself now, you'll have to make time to be sick later. Allow yourself to reach your full potential and be your very best. Eat Bulletproof. Be Bulletproof.

CHAPTER 2

BULLETPROOFING YOUR FOOD

It's relatively simple to make food that tastes good. It's also simple enough to make food that's supposed to be healthy but that doesn't taste good. But being Bulletproof is all about making food that gives you a natural energy high and tastes great. Generally speaking, food that makes you feel good, food that you enjoy, tastes good to you. The brain likes it, so you crave it. You may create a food high by using ingredients and preparations that satisfy in the short term, but weigh you down and sap energy. Bulletproof eating means finding the right foods and preparing them in a way that leaves you buzzing with energy. I recommend a blend of high fat, moderate protein, and tons of veggies, using ingredients that won't cause food cravings.

The best part is that Bulletproof eating is delicious and gratifying. My all-time favorite food is grass-fed rib-eye. I also happen to believe that every food tastes better with a spoonful of guacamole on top, made with lots of tasty, fatty avocados. When I'm preparing vegetables—any kind at all—I steam or blanch them, then take a third of the portion and blend it with butter and Bulletproof Brain Octane oil. Then I mix that puree back in with the rest of the veggies. It's like eating creamed spinach, but honestly, even better because you're getting so much nutritional benefit. So you can see, my favored style of eating is anything but boring or bland. Bulletproof eating should also curtail your desire to snack. When you're eating this way, your body stays satisfied until the next mealtime. That said, if you do experience a snack craving, I recommend salmon and avocado or a little bit of very dark chocolate with high cacao content.

You can see the entire Bulletproof Roadmap at www.bulletproof.com/diet-roadmap-poster, which graphically breaks down the best and worst foods for building energy. But let's look at categories of food as you might in a grocery store. I'd like to give you some rules of the road for choosing different food types when you're making a decision at the butcher counter or the veggie bins.

FATS

There's a lot of misinformation about fats—which ones to eat and in what amounts. This section will detail how to choose the optimal fats for becoming bulletproof.

HEALTHY FATS

The Fat Scare that started in the 1970s convinced people that saturated fats were detrimental to their health, and that they should be avoided at all costs. That information was based on terrible science, and the idea that saturated fats are linked to heart disease has since been debunked. Saturated fats are not associated with cardiovascular disease—trans fats and polyunsaturated omega-6 fats are. Fats are necessary for proper cell functioning and metabolism, and are the building blocks for cell membranes and hormones. It is essential that you get enough healthy fats in your diet in order to perform well, both physically and mentally. However, it is also important to know that not all fats are created equal. Canola oil from GMO corn and butter made from sick, grain-fed cows are not the same as cold-pressed, organic extra virgin olive oil, medium-chain triglyceride (MCT) oil from organic coconut and palm, or butter from cows that have eaten their natural diet of grass their entire life!

When I talk about fats, I'm referring to those derived from animal sources, like meat, fish, and dairy. When you're eating Bulletproof, one of the most important things you can do is to ensure that your body gets raw or undamaged fats. See, fats are very delicate. They are easily ruined by heat, light, or oxygen, which strips them of their nutrient content.

While you can get your necessary good fat content from coconut oil or ghee, the best possible source is fat from grass-fed local animals. This fat is going to be nutrient-dense—unless you cook it at too high a temperature, like 500°F, and ruin it. When you're cooking meat (beef and lamb in particular), there's a great temptation—and one advised by many chefs—to sear the meat before cooking it through. However, frying damages fats through oxidation and makes them hard for your body to metabolize and use.

The searing of meat is what's known as the maillard reaction, the process of browning meat not only to change the color and create a textural crust, but actually to change the chemical compound of the meat and affect the flavor, bringing out that rich, umami flavor. Umami flavor is deeply satisfying, but because these flavors come from glutamic acid or monosodium glutamate (MSG)—which causes a blood sugar drop resulting in food cravings—umami foods can

cause more cravings after ingestion. So while it's true that the maillard reaction does lock in the juices and create an umami flavor profile, searing also destroys those precious fats by changing their molecular structure. You need to be careful with heat, time, air, and light, treating those fats gently. What I recommend is adding that patina at the end of the cooking cycle, rather than shocking and damaging the fats at the beginning.

I recommend cooking beef and lamb gently or with moisture, like in a sous-vide. I recommend lower heat for more time so fats cook gently. Then you can quickly brown them at the end.

This same approach holds true for salmon, a beautiful form of precious omega-3 fats, and one of my favorite sources. Many of us understand that salmon and other fish are chock full of these "good fats," but the way the salmon is prepared or cured has a great effect on whether you're getting the nutritional benefits or not. Omega-3s are fragile, and damaging them is actually highly inflammatory to the body. This is especially true with hot-smoked salmon, which uses a process linked to cancer-causing carcinogens. Hot-smoked salmon is cured with—you guessed it—hot smoke, resulting in far more oxidized fats and the formation of problematic compounds. On the other hand, cold-smoked salmon is superhealthy because it's cured with salt and refrigerated with liquid smoke so its fats remain intact and aren't damaged by the smoking process. If you're planning to cook fresh salmon, poach it, steam it, or gently bake it. The goal is to keep those gorgeous fats in perfect shape.

Grass-Fed Butter

Commercially raised dairy cows are fed grains (and all manner of other unthinkable things) because grains are cheaper and more calorie dense. This allows farms to fit more cows into a smaller space, which is great for producing more food, but terrible for the cows' health. These living conditions require the use of antibiotics to keep the cows from getting sick, but to make matters worse, the grains that the cows feed on are typically stored in poor fashion, and are easily contaminated with mold. The mold in the grains produces toxins that are ingested by the cows and stored in their fats, which are

WHY SHOULD YOU USE BRAIN OCTANE OIL INSTEAD OF REGULAR MCT OR COCONUT OIL IN MY RECIPES?

It's pretty simple, really. Brain Octane is 100 percent medium-chain triglycerides (MCTs). The coconut oil industry would have you believe that there are four kinds of MCT oils found in coconut oil: C6, C8, C10, and C12 (lauric acid) (the numbers define the length of the carbon chains). But, really, only a small amount of the coconut oil is actually MCT. While it's true that these are all called MCTs, we now know that C12, or lauric acid, is actually a pseudo-MCT.

Lauric acid is actually a good food source, but it acts like an LCT (long-chain triglyceride) rather than an MCT when you consume it, so you don't get the fast ketone energy from it that you can get from C8 or C10. Lauric acid also doesn't get processed in the body in the same way as true MCTs. It still has to go through a breakdown process in the liver, which takes longer and uses more bodily resources. So while coconut oil is a food that we like, it's not your most Bulletproof option. My recipes are designed and written to give you the very best performance.

So, when you're looking for quick energy and you want to convert those fats to ketones, why would you choose a diluted version when you could get more bang for your buck? If you use Brain Octane oil, the whole amount will be converted to energy quickly, while only a small amount of the coconut oil can offer that same benefit.

then passed on to humans in their beef and dairy products. The fat in the cows also contains higher amounts of inflammatory omega-6 fatty acids due to the high omega-6 content of the grains they eat. Grass-fed cows are much healthier because they are eating the food that nature intended them to eat, and they also avoid the toxins and molds found in commercial feeds. Grass-fed cows produce far higher quality meat and dairy products that contain a different fat and nutrient profile, with higher amounts of omega-3 fatty acids, and beneficial compounds like conjugated linoleic acid (CLA) and butyrate (butyric acid). CLA has anti-cancer benefits and weight-loss uses, while butyrate helps heal the gut and turn off brain inflammation.

You may also choose to use ghee, a type of clarified butter. Ghee has some benefits over butter in that the milk protein, casein, is removed in the making of ghee. It also has a higher smoke point than butter, so it's preferable for use as a cooking agent as it won't burn as easily.

Krill Oil

Similar to fish oil, krill oil comes from tiny shrimp and is a rich source of the polyunsaturated omega-3 fatty acids, EPA (eicosapentaenoic acid) and DHA (docosahexaenoic acid). EPA and DHA are considered "nutritionally essential" because they are required in order for your body (and particularly your brain) to function properly, yet we cannot make them on our own and must ingest them from foods. DHA plays a central role in the function of synaptic connections in the brain, and your brain and nervous system are so dependent on this compound that any deficiencies can lead to degenerative disorders, such as Alzheimer's disease, multiple sclerosis, schizophrenia, dementia, and depression. Omega-3 fatty acids provide other important benefits as well, including reduction of inflammation, possibly improvement of muscle growth, and, according to some studies, treatment of PMS.

Krill oil is the preferred source of EPA and DHA because the polyunsaturated fats are packaged as phospholipids, which can be easily absorbed and integrated in the body. The EPA and DHA in fish oil are usually packaged as triglycerides, and must undergo additional processing in order to be utilized properly. Flax oil also contains omega-3 fats, however much of it comes in the form of alpha-linolenic acid (ALA). Our bodies can convert ALA into DHA, but only at a rate of 1 percent to 4 percent—a woefully low conversion rate. Krill oil also contains the powerful antioxidant astaxanthin, which helps to

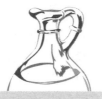

Oil & Fats

BULLETPROOF ▲

Bulletproof Brain Octane, Bulletproof MCT Oil, Bulletproof Ghee, Bulletproof Chocolate, Bulletproof Cocoa Butter, pastured egg yolks†, krill oil, grass-fed red meat fat and marrow, avocado oil, coconut oil, sunflower lecithin

fish oil, grass-fed butter and ghee

palm oil, palm kernel, pastured bacon fat, raw macadamias, extra virgin olive oil

raw almonds, hazelnuts, walnuts, cashew butter, non-GMO soy lecithin

duck and goose fat, grain-fed butter and ghee

factory chicken fat; safflower, sunflower, canola, peanut, soy, cottonseed, corn, and vegetable oils; heated nuts and oils; flaxseed oil

margarine and other artificial trans fats, oils made from GMO grains, commercial lard

KRYPTONITE ▼

† Verify that you are not allergic to eggs.

Download your color copy at www.bulletproof.com/diet-roadmap-poster

protect the fragile omega-3 fats from breaking down since they are so unstable. It makes a wonderful supplement to any Bulletproof plan.

Coconut Oil and Medium-Chain Triglyceride (MCT) Oil

Coconut has been used as a food staple and medicine by many different cultures throughout history. Coconut oil is a source of many healthy fats, is high in fiber, and also acts as a powerful natural antibiotic, virucide, fungicide, and parasiticide. Coconut oil has devastating effects on viruses, bacteria, parasites, and microorganisms that cause many disorders, including ulcers, cavities, urinary tract infections, and more, but it doesn't harm the probiotic flora that populate your gut and intestinal tract.

MCT oil is a type of saturated fat found in tropical plants, such as coconut or palm, and is responsible for many of the health benefits associated with those foods. There are two types of MCTs: caprylic acid and capric acid, both of which are converted immediately into energy by your body without requiring any processing in the liver like other, longer-chain fats. These fats are converted into ketone bodies, an alternate type of energy that is used by your brain. MCT oil not only provides that quick burst of energy, but also promotes healthy cholesterol levels. It's tasteless and odorless, which makes it incredibly easy to integrate into your diet. It's just a flavorless liquid you can drizzle onto your food, use as salad dressing, or add to smoothies. Plus, you can heat it up to 320°F and still enjoy the health benefits.

Extra Virgin Olive Oil

Olives are a great source of monounsaturated fats, which help to optimize cholesterol levels, particularly beneficial HDL cholesterol, and have been linked to lower risk of heart disease. Olive oil also has a host of other benefits, including assisting with blood clotting, regulating blood sugars, and promoting insulin sensitivity; and it contains several powerful polyphenols that act as antioxidants and anti-inflammatory agents. Some studies have even shown that olive oil can reduce the risk of several types of cancer and slow cognitive decline. It is important to use "extra virgin," since plain and light olive oil both contain far fewer polyphenols. And you should check the label to make sure that it is pure 100 percent olive oil and doesn't contain any additives or filler oils. Since olive oil is not saturated, it is fairly unstable and easy to oxidize, and you should never cook with it. Any amount of heat will start to oxidize the oil, which can create inflammatory free radicals. Stick to using your oil on salads or cold sauces. Make sure to buy a brand that comes in a dark glass container to limit the amount of light exposure, and use the oil within a year of buying to ensure it hasn't gone rancid.

FATS TO AVOID

Not all fats are created equal, and there are many fats, including some that have a ridiculous "heart-healthy" label, that are detrimental to your health and should be avoided whenever possible.

Seed, Soy, and Vegetable Oils

All of these types of oils are extremely high in inflammatory omega-6 fatty acids. We do need a little bit of omega-6 in order to function properly, but the Standard American Diet (SAD) includes way too many of these oils, and the ratio of omega-6 to omega-3 oils is far too high, resulting in rampant inflammation. On top of that, omega-6s oxidize very easily and go rancid when cooked, resulting in free radicals that cause even more inflammation in the body. For this reason, many of these oils are hydrogenated and converted into trans fats to increase their stability. These Franken-fats have been shown to drastically increase LDL cholesterol levels and increase the risk for heart disease. Combine all of that with the fact that many of these oils come from GMO crops and foods that are typically contaminated with mycotoxins, and there are plenty of reasons to avoid them.

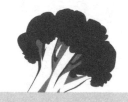

Organic Veggies

asparagus, avocado,
bok choy*, broccoli*,
brussels sprouts*, cauliflower,
celery, cucumber, fennel,
olives

cabbage*, collards*, kale*,
lettuce, radishes, spinach*,
summer squash, zucchini

artichokes, butternut and
winter squash, carrots, green
beans, green onion, leeks,
parsley

eggplant, onion, peas,
peppers, shallots, tomatoes

beets, mushrooms, pumpkin,
raw chard, raw collards, raw
kale, raw spinach

corn (fresh on the cob)

all other corn except fresh,
canned veggies, soy

* These items should be cooked. Refer to
Chapter 3 for the most Bulletproof way of
preparing these veggies.

Download your color copy at www.bulletproof.com/diet-roadmap-poster

The vegetable-based omega-3s found in oils like flax and hemp are converted by our bodies into beneficial DHA at a very inefficient rate, so it is better to stick with other sources and avoid the high–omega-6 content.

Commercial Lard

Much like the difference between the dairy from grain-fed and grass-fed cows, the lard produced from commercial cows contains hormones and antibiotics, and has a fat profile that is high in omega-6 fats and lacking in beneficial omega-3s, CLA, and butyric acid. Stick to using healthy saturated fats like coconut oil and grass-fed butter. That said, if you can find local, organic, nonhydrogenated lard, that would be fine.

VEGETABLES

If you've looked at the Bulletproof Roadmap, you've gathered that I recommend a whole lot of vegetables in your daily diet. When you're shopping for veggies, my rule of thumb is to go for organic, followed by fresh (which really means local, so you have less transportation time involved from harvesting to your table). Organic foods come to you just as nature intended them, bursting with all the nutrients your body craves. So organic plus fresh is ideal. Organic and less fresh is OK, but perhaps slightly less nutrient-rich. If you can't get organic, a good option is local, fresh, and unsprayed. Please be sure foods called fresh actually are because nonorganic foods can be plumped or dyed to look fresh when they're not. They can also be pumped full of nasty chemicals and pesticides, so again, I say no thanks. I'd rather have a bedraggled-looking organic item than a shiny non-organic one.

MEATS

For optimal Bulletproof eating, you want to get a moderate amount of super-high-quality protein. Getting high-quality produce and meats is essential for ensuring that you're feeding your body good nutrients and avoiding harmful toxins and additives. Grass-fed beef and lamb, wild-caught fish, and pastured pork are all things you should be striving to eat as much as possible. Some people complain that high-quality foods are too expensive, but if you consider the illness and medical bills associated with eating low-nutrient foods for an extended period of time, taking care of yourself and eating well is actually the more cost-effective approach—and you'll have the benefit of better health and quality of life.

CHICKEN: NOT YOUR BEST BULLETPROOF CHOICE

One of the biggest misconceptions I encounter is that chicken is a dieter's best friend.

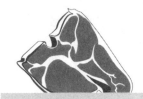

Protein

BULLETPROOF

Bulletproof Whey, Bulletproof Collagen Protein, Bulletproof CollaGelatin, grass-fed beef and lamb, pastured eggs† and gelatin, colostrum

low-mercury wild fish such as anchovies, haddock, petrale sole, sardines, sockeye salmon, summer flounder, trout

pastured pork, clean whey isolate*, pastured duck and goose

factory-farmed eggs†, pastured chicken and turkey

heated whey, hemp protein, factory-farmed meat

high-mercury or farmed seafood, rice, and pea protein

KRYPTONITE

soy protein, wheat protein, beans, cheese, and other pasteurized or cooked dairy (except butter)

* Whey protein should be cold processed and cross-flow microfiltered (CFM). People who are sensitive to dairy should use isolate over concentrate.

† Verify that you are not allergic to eggs.

Download your color copy at www.bulletproof.com/diet-roadmap-poster

The thing is, lean chicken breast can raise insulin almost like sugar, and skin-on breast has polyunsaturated fat. So, there are far better sources for you to get both your protein and your fat than chicken. Grass-fed lamb or beef is going to offer far better fatty acid composition without the insulin spike. Plus, if you're concerned about cruelty-free choices, grass-fed beef better supports our ecology.

Believe me, I tried to find a chicken I could get behind. I searched the world for the best heritage chicken anywhere. You can feed chickens coconuts, but their fat will still be polyunsaturated, which is not ideal for Bulletproof results. Another thing people don't know is that chickens are carnivorous. They like to eat critters, but most farm-raised chickens are fed veggie food, so they're actually malnourished. Any chicken farmer can attest to this, and my own experience raising a rooster named Hannibal bore this out. So really, if an animal is not nourished, how can their flesh be a nutrient source that makes you feel your best? If you're going to find chicken, you'll want it local and free range, just be prepared to pay a bit more for the quality you're getting.

GRASS-FED AND GRASS-FINISHED MEATS

If you choose high-quality beef or lamb, you'll want to make sure it's not only grass-fed, but also grass-finished. Most people don't realize that in order for meat to be labeled grass-fed, that doesn't mean 100 percent of the time. Some ranchers feed animals grain in the latter part of their lives, which is important because it changes the composition of the meat's nutrient offering. So be sure that you're looking for beef or lamb that is grass-finished as well as grass-fed. If you can't find grass-finished or grass-fed meat, choose the leanest cuts of grain-fed meat possible. If you *can* find grass-fed meat—choose the fattiest cuts possible.

GO FOR FRESH FLAVOR

The next thing to consider when choosing meat is whether or not it's fresh and local. These days, foodies are all about dry-aged beef because of its deep umami flavor. However, that process actually involves hanging the beef and growing a fungus on it, which is later cut off. I'll admit, this process creates nice flavor and tender texture, but those fungi also produce mold toxins that cause food cravings. So I say no thanks. When you're looking to eat Bulletproof and feel your energetic best, you don't want meat that's been hung and aged or transported a long way—you want it fresh and local.

Another reason to think local is that more and more ranchers these days are using genetically modified (GMO) grass, which is grown and mowed somewhere offsite and brought onsite. GMO grass is not only bad for you, it's also simply less nutritious. So look for grass-fed and grass-finished meat that is grown locally and sold fresh. That's the best you can do in this department. And if you have to pick between grass-fed and organic, go grass-fed. That's because organic meat that's not grass-fed can be fed moldy corn and soy, as long as they are organic. You don't want grain-fed meat, even if the grains are organic!

PORK

I know we've all heard that pork is "the other white meat," with the connotation that it's healthy for us, but when you're eating Bulletproof, grass-fed red meats are a far superior choice. Pigs are foragers that eat garbage, so their flesh is teeming with parasites. Also, pig farmers will often feed pigs whatever they can to fatten them up. In the most egregious cases, that can mean actual garbage or even dead animals. Now, if you get pastured pigs, that eliminates a lot of the issue, so pastured is the key if you like to eat pork. Also, if you plan to eat bacon, you should look for a variety with no added nitrates. There are methods by which you can actually cure bacon using natural ingredients like celery, and that process will produce nitrates naturally, so that's going to be a better option

than the chemicals that companies add to their bacon.

DAIRY

Let me state this clearly and simply: You should avoid most dairy protein. Dairy is full of casein, phosphoproteins that are common in mammalian milk. Casein triggers inflammation, causes allergies in many people, and also makes you experience more cravings. (Have you ever noticed that it's hard to stop eating cheese? Blame the casein.) Although casein isn't great for you, milk is actually an excellent source of fat. In a perfect world, we'd all have raw, local, grass-fed, whole milk with which to make butter. But that type of milk—and butter made from it—is very expensive. It's a luxury food. That's why I look to grass-fed meats and grass-fed (but not necessarily raw) butter for my proteins and fats. And I recommend a high-quality grass-fed whey protein powder (like Bulletproof) as a great source of the good stuff.

If you're interested in dairy substitutes, you should consider almond milk, ideally homemade. Most commercially processed varieties are highly processed with bad stuff and depleted of nutrients. And it's so easy to make it at home with good-quality raw almonds, hot water, a blender, and cheesecloth. It tastes great and the fats won't be

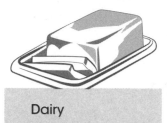

Dairy

BULLETPROOF ▲

Bulletproof Ghee, organic grass-fed butter, colostrum

nonorganic grass-fed ghee or butter, organic grass-fed cream

organic grass-fed full-fat raw milk or yogurt

nonorganic grass-fed ghee or butter, organic grass-fed cream

grain-fed butter

skim or low-fat milk, fake butter, pasteurized nonorganic milk or yogurt

all cheese, powdered milk, factory dairy, dairy replacer, condensed or evaporated milk, conventional ice cream

▼ KRYPTONITE

Dairy protein is a major source of allergies and inflammation. Test yourself to see what works. Ghee is safe for almost everyone, and butter usually is too because it is low in protein.

Download your color copy at www.bulletproof.com/diet-roadmap-poster

damaged by this simple process. Cashew milk is OK, but it tends to have more sugar, so I recommend almonds if you're going the nut milk route. You should steer clear of soy milk entirely. It's always a bad idea because it inhibits thyroid function and contains inflammatory omega-6 fats and excessive estrogen. Also, most of it is GMO so it contains glyphosate residues. Just say no to soy.

FRUITS

Many people striving to eat healthy put fruits and vegetables in the same category, but fruits are nowhere near as beneficial as veggies from a Bulletproof standpoint. Fruits have a large concentration of sugars. That said, not all fruits are created equal. I prefer berries because they are low in sugar and high in antioxidants. But if there's one fruit I swear by, it's that rarely-recognized-as-fruit— avocado. It's a perfect source of fats, and it's delicious with everything. Did I mention that I will put guacamole on pretty much anything? It's definitely one of my favorite choices for nutritional value and flavor.

GRAINS

Let's talk about grains. Contrary to popular opinion, I'm not antigrain for some trendy "carbs are evil" reason. I'm antigrain because grains have natural defenses that aren't beneficial to us. Think of it this way: A grain's whole job—its *raison d'être*—is to sprout new plants. So, through evolution, grains have developed natural defenses to keep predators from eating them. And guess what? Those predators also include humans. All whole grains contain antinutrients to discourage animals from eating them.

The other issue with grains is about storage. Grain storage leads to mold growth, a problem that we think of as belonging only to the Third World, but it's true of grain storage in North America as well. My research reveals that a little mold toxin can make you tired and cranky and, according to multiple studies, can damage your DNA. It's such a problem that levels of some mycotoxins—but not others—are limited by governments. Different governments differ on safe levels, and even "safe" levels are not beneficial. It's interesting to note that 85 percent of people with Crohn's disease have tested positive for a type of mold toxin called aflatoxin. Chronic gut problems are often associated with mycotoxins in food, a little known fact. Just another reason I'm not a fan of eating foods that contain these mold chemicals.

If you're going to eat grains, it's helpful to know that white rice is the least problematic, followed by quinoa. Many people believe brown rice is superior, but it's irritating to the

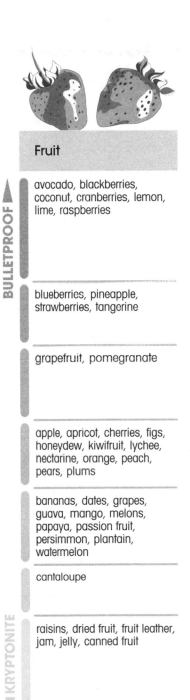

Fruit

BULLETPROOF ▲

avocado, blackberries, coconut, cranberries, lemon, lime, raspberries

blueberries, pineapple, strawberries, tangerine

grapefruit, pomegranate

apple, apricot, cherries, figs, honeydew, kiwifruit, lychee, nectarine, orange, peach, pears, plums

bananas, dates, grapes, guava, mango, melons, papaya, passion fruit, persimmon, plantain, watermelon

cantaloupe

▼ KRYPTONITE

raisins, dried fruit, fruit leather, jam, jelly, canned fruit

BRAIN-BOOSTING SUPPLEMENTS

Healthy fats aren't the only thing you can add to your diet in order to boost your intelligence. There are other food-based supplements available that you can integrate into your lifestyle to help protect your brain health and optimize mental performance.

Acetyl L-Carnitine (ALCAR)

ALCAR is an amino acid that acts as an antioxidant in the brain. ALCAR has been shown to enhance the effects of acetylcholine, a stimulating neurotransmitter, to help your brain work better. It also enhances the function of dopamine, the neurotransmitter responsible for reward and pleasure feelings in your brain, and acts as a powerful cognitive enhancer. Recent research has also demonstrated that ALCAR can help to increase fat oxidation in your mitochondria, the energy powerhouses in your cells. It's sold in capsules and powder form, with dosages recommended on the label.

Oxaloacetate

A naturally occurring supplement found in every cell in your body, oxaloacetate has many benefits, including all the benefits that research has shown are associated with caloric restriction, like improvements in aging. However, the most important benefit is that it protects your brain from damage by reducing harmful glutamate levels. Glutamate is the most common neurotransmitter in your body and an excessive build-up can be toxic and cause all manner of problems, including cognitive impairment, sleep problems, stress, and even cell death from excitation. Oxaloacetate protects your brain and mitochondria so that you aren't hampered by brain fog and mental fatigue. My own product that is rich in oxaloacetate is called Upgraded Aging Formula.

Creatine

Typically associated with sports and athletic performance supplements, creatine has actually been shown to have powerful brain-boosting effects too! Studies have shown that creatine can boost cognitive performance, and that there can even be a small IQ boost for those in their 30s who take it daily. It's also good for those under 30 and even great for anyone over 40.

gut and contains approximately 80 times more arsenic than white rice, which is why white rice is the only grain I suggest. There are plenty of other great sources of foods that give you valuable nutrients without all the negative effects. If you're going to eat grains, I've listed them on this page from most favorable to least.

STARCHES

There's quite a bit of controversy about starches because of their glucose content, but they also have supernutrient components, and your body can benefit from some starch. Starches are fine in moderation, unless you're trying to be in ketosis. However, you want ones that aren't going to spike your blood sugar a lot, and ones that will feed your gut bacteria, like those listed on this page in my order of preference.

NUTS

Nuts are subject to many spoilage-based toxins because of their sourcing and their storage, so I'm choosy about the ones I'll use and I eat them in moderation. Choose raw, organic nuts from the list on page 34 and keep them sealed in the fridge or, for some nuts, freezing is OK. The list includes nuts in my order of preference.

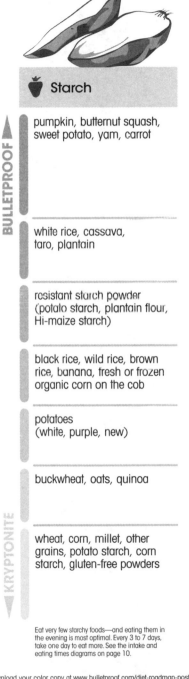

Starch

BULLETPROOF

pumpkin, butternut squash, sweet potato, yam, carrot

white rice, cassava, taro, plantain

resistant starch powder (potato starch, plantain flour, Hi-maize starch)

black rice, wild rice, brown rice, banana, fresh or frozen organic corn on the cob

potatoes (white, purple, new)

buckwheat, oats, quinoa

KRYPTONITE

wheat, corn, millet, other grains, potato starch, corn starch, gluten-free powders

Eat very few starchy foods—and eating them in the evening is most optimal. Every 3 to 7 days, take one day to eat more. See the intake and eating times diagrams on page 10.

Download your color copy at www.bulletproof.com/diet-roadmap-poster

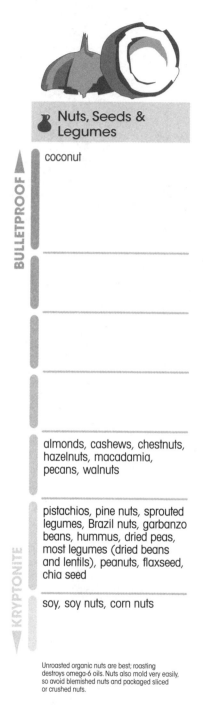

Nuts, Seeds & Legumes

BULLETPROOF ↑

coconut

---

almonds, cashews, chestnuts, hazelnuts, macadamia, pecans, walnuts

pistachios, pine nuts, sprouted legumes, Brazil nuts, garbanzo beans, hummus, dried peas, most legumes (dried beans and lentils), peanuts, flaxseed, chia seed

soy, soy nuts, corn nuts

↓ KRYPTONITE

Unroasted organic nuts are best; roasting destroys omega-6 oils. Nuts also mold very easily, so avoid blemished nuts and packaged sliced or crushed nuts.

Download your color copy at www.bulletproof.com/diet-roadmap-poster

VINEGARS AND PICKLED THINGS

If you're someone who likes strong, tangy tastes, as many people do, be thoughtful about where you find them. Apple cider vinegar is a good choice for health purposes because it doesn't have many yeast or grain toxins, unlike other vinegars. Exotic vinegars like balsamic, red wine, or champagne varieties almost always contain inflammation-causing yeast toxins, hidden sugars, and heavy metals.

Likewise, pickles also run the gamut. Pickles can be naturally fermented and full of probiotics or they can be full of sugar. They can be naturally fermented with a controlled healthy probiotic culture, or growing strange wild bacteria in a bucket. As with everything else, the mantra here is purity. Normally, you get that from fresh and local, but with fermentation, the trick is to work with someone—ideally someone local, but far away, if necessary—who is using controlled cultures to make fermented foods with known healthy probiotics, not wild yeast. Know who makes your pickled product, or better yet, make it yourself. Avoid products with lots of preservatives and ingredients you can't pronounce.

HERBS AND SPICES

Variety is the spice of life. Or maybe spice is the variety of life? When it comes to Bulletproof eating, spices are important for both health reasons and great flavor. Most herbs and spices are good for you on some level. Many have antioxidant properties and others have specific benefits, like helping digestion. But some really knock it out of the park when it comes to nutrition and wellness.

I use spices, herbs, and other flavorings to maximize flavor as well as performance. You may not realize just how powerful some spices are in keeping your body running optimally by bolstering immunity or offering antiseptic properties. I'll share the ones that offer the most benefit while minimizing exposure to antinutrients and keeping you on track while biohacking your body.

Part of the way you become more Bulletproof starts in your gut. It's the root of your health and it can affect all your other bodily systems. So in order to start healing your gut and developing healthy gut flora, the idea is to eat actively anti-inflammatory foods since inflammation is the cause of many chronic diseases. Inflammation can occur on the cellular level in one or more body systems, and reducing it is the first step to biohacking your body. Until you do this, you can't really perform at optimal levels and you can't feel your physical or mental best.

When your body isn't inflamed anymore, you'll know it because you'll feel lighter, brighter, more vibrant—and you won't feel that muffin top hanging over your waistband

either. Sometimes we have that extra flab because of excess weight, but it's often due to inflammation (literally swelling) in the belly.

Spices aren't the only food group that helps treat inflammation: Dark leafy greens and cruciferous vegetables like broccoli and cabbage are wonderful antioxidants, as are omega-3–rich fish, egg yolks, and grass-fed meats. However, I'm going to focus right now on spices because, ounce for ounce, herbs and spices pack a potent punch compared to other anti-inflammatory foods. You'd be amazed what adding a few carefully preserved and treated herbs and veggies can go to amplify the power—and the flavor—of almost any meal.

As with anything I eat, I like to preserve spices in their natural form as much as possible. I recommend finding spices in their whole form and grinding them yourself if at all possible. Some spices have specific utensils like a nutmeg grater, but you can also use a coffee grinder to crush spices if you like. Herbs are often best in their raw state, chopped and sprinkled over foods or only very lightly cooked. Let their natural flavor shine through and preserve the nutrients in their essential form for best results.

IT ALL STARTS WITH AYURVEDA

Traditional Chinese Medicine and the Indian tradition of Ayurveda, both ancient systems of Eastern medicine, have known about the healing properties of herbs and spices for centuries.

They still use them today to treat all kinds of ailments, from digestion to migraines to menopause. Because herbs and spices are rich in antioxidants, they help fend off free radicals that damage cells and lead to inflammation. These nutrients can also halt genes that trigger inflammatory proteins or processes. Suffice it to say, spices are your friend. And just so you get a picture of how potent they are, think about this: Just ½ teaspoon of ground cinnamon has as many antioxidants as ½ cup blueberries, and ½ teaspoon dried oregano has the antioxidant power of 3 cups of raw spinach.

So, on the opposite page, in order of most beneficial, are the top Bulletproof herbs and spices.

Turmeric

Turmeric is the king of all spices. Ounce for ounce, it's the most anti-inflammatory, antiviral, antibacterial, anticancer, antifungal one of the bunch, so you should eat it as much as possible when you're becoming Bulletproof. In Ayurveda and Traditional Chinese Medicine, it's used to treat everything from diabetes and allergies to Alzheimer's and arthritis. Turmeric's active ingredient is curcumin, an antioxidant compound that reduces inflammation and also gives it its vibrant yellow color. (Beware getting turmeric on anything white; it stains.) Curcumin has actually been shown to reduce growth in cancer cells, and

if there's any good reason to eat a spice, I'd say that's it. Turmeric also contains other anti-inflammatory compounds that inhibit swelling and pain and block the plaques that cause Alzheimer's disease. So the takeaway is? Eat more turmeric. Add it to salad dressings, meat and fish marinades, or even turmeric-infused tea, latte, or lemonade. It's surprisingly tasty.

Chile Peppers and Cayenne

Cayenne's active ingredient is capsaicin, which delivers both a chile pepper's medicinal qualities and its spicy heat. The hotter a pepper, the more capsaicin it has. In addition to a long history of medicinal uses in India and China, Native American healers favored cayenne for digestive and circulatory problems. For all its good benefits though, there are some negative aspects of capsaicin. Like black pepper, cayenne is highly likely to have high amounts of mold toxins, so proper sourcing and storage is really key. I do make notes in my recipes about where and how to use it, but just keep that caution in mind. Sourced and stored properly, cayenne is a fantastic source of antioxidants that fight free radicals and protect against cell damage, which often manifests as premature aging. There are promising studies underway to observe whether cayenne inhibits cancer cell growth, but the science is still young.

Ginger

Ginger has long been used in Ayurveda and Traditional Chinese Medicine to combat inflammation and pain, soothe sore muscles, and treat aches and fatigue. It's also a common remedy for digestion as it fights an overgrowth of nasty gut bacteria. The compounds in ginger actually act in a similar way to anti-inflammatory drugs, like ibuprofen, that are used to treat arthritis. If more people knew this, more people might be able to find relief from ginger tea or Asian dishes. Ginger is also great for sore throats, colds, and believe it or not, you can apply it directly to a painful joint with a compress for relief through skin contact.

As with all spices and herbs, storage is important for ginger. Poorly stored ginger powder is at risk for mycotoxin contamination and fresh ginger can get moldy in the fridge. So while I want you to use and eat ginger regularly, buy it fresh, use it up, and toss the stuff that's been hanging around. Or, if you go the powdered route (which won't be as potent), be sure to store it someplace away from heat, light, and moisture. If you decide to cook with ginger and you're using oil, add it at the end of cooking because, cooked with fat, it can get a bitter taste. Also, if you like ginger with your sushi, go for the yellow variety. The pink stuff you

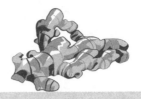

Spices & Flavorings

BULLETPROOF ▲

Bulletproof Chocolate Powder, Bulletproof Vanillamax, apple cider vinegar, cilantro, coffee*, ginger*, parsley, sea salt

lavender, oregano, rosemary, thyme, turmeric

allspice, cinnamon, cloves*, organic prepared mustard with no additives

mustard seed, onion, table salt

black pepper*, conventional chocolate, garlic*, nutmeg*, paprika*

miso, tamari, tofu

KRYPTONITE ▼

commercial dressings, spice mixes and extracts, MSG, yeast, caseinate, textured protein, bouillon and broth, hydrolyzed gluten, anything labeled enzyme-modified flavoring or seasoning

* Beware, these items often harbor toxic mold species. It's best to use fresh, high-quality options whenever you can.

Download your color copy at www.bulletproof.com/diet-roadmap-poster

see in some restaurants has been colored with an artificial dye. Both kinds have sugar, but the yellow stuff is preferable.

Cinnamon

Cinnamon is most touted for its ability to lower blood sugar in people with diabetes. As with its spicy counterparts, cinnamon contains compounds with antioxidant and anti-inflammatory properties that reduce the likelihood of cellular damage and chronic disease. It's been shown to protect against heart disease by preventing blood platelets from clumping and to inhibit abnormal cell growth, making it a powerful anticancer option.

Cloves

Cloves are a rich source of antioxidants that scavenge free radicals and help protect cells. They are also a powerful antifungal in the body, whether ingested or applied topically. Beware, though, clove oil is potent stuff. It's so strong it can be toxic if overused. I recommend using whole cloves whenever possible.

Sage

You won't be surprised to learn that sage, too, has anti-inflammatory molecules, which contribute to its flavor and aroma. Sage is specifically thought to protect against inflammation-based neurological conditions, like Alzheimer's, and it shows promise for improving memory and concentration at the same time. Its compounds also have antioxidant and anticancer effects. Packed with camphor, its extracts can be used to kill bacteria and fungi, so it's a powerful spice when eaten, or used in a natural kitchen cleaning solution.

Rosemary

Like sage, rosemary contains antioxidant and anti-inflammatory compounds. It

GINGER COMPRESS

A ginger compress can be used to treat arthritis or common colds. To make a simple compress, start by bringing water to a boil and then reducing to a simmer and dropping in a golf ball–size sachet of finely chopped ginger. Let it steep for 5 minutes and then dip small towels in the water and apply to a sore area or the chest for a cold, covering it with another towel to retain heat. Continue dipping, wringing, and pressing the towel against the area for 15 to 20 minutes.

increases the activity of an enzyme that removes free radicals associated with chronic inflammation. This is especially true when the herb is cooked, so add it liberally to vegetables, meats, and other savory cooked dishes. You can use it raw too, as the flavonoids in rosemary have been shown to inhibit the growth of pancreatic cancer cells and prevent hemorrhoids. A hint about using rosemary: If you're going to cook something in oil, add some rosemary and it will help prevent detrimental oxidation to the oil because rosmarinic acid is an antioxidant.

But What about Black Pepper?

People often ask why black pepper isn't on the list, and no, it's not an oversight. While black pepper can increase the absorption of turmeric, it's very hard to find it without aflatoxin, which is the most potent mycotoxin of them all. I'd rather avoid the mycotoxin in black pepper than hope for a benefit from what may or may not be a tainted source.

HOW TO STORE YOUR SPICES TO AVOID MOLD

Mold can grow just about anywhere, from the counter to the fridge. And while you've probably seen a moldy sprig of herbs in the vegetable drawer before, you may not have considered that spices mold easily too. Spices are often irradiated to prevent this spoilage, which means radiation is used to sterilize them. That may kill the likelihood of mold, but it also kills some of the nutrient and antioxidant power of spices—just as microwaving food can kill its nutritional composition. While irradiating the spices may prevent some molds, it's not a failsafe method, and there's another factor to consider as well. Picture this: You reach up into the spice cabinet to grab some paprika and sprinkle it over your steamy pan of Hungarian chicken. When you open the canister and shake out some spice, a warm, moist mist of steam enters the spice canister, only to be sealed up and tucked back in the warm cabinet above the stove. Welcome, mold spores; we've found your perfect home. The best thing you can do to increase your performance and not subject yourself to these inferior and potentially mold-ridden spices is to toss opened, old spices that are more than a couple months old. (I bet some of you would be embarrassed to admit how many *years* old some of your spices are.) Starting now, make an effort to use only high-quality, recently opened, fresh or dried herbs and spices or, if you can't commit to that, don't use them at all.

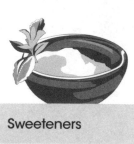

Sweeteners

BULLETPROOF

xylitol, erythritol, stevia

sorbitol, maltitol, and other sugar alcohols

non-GMO dextrose, glucose, raw honey

maple syrup, coconut sugar

white sugar, brown sugar, agave, cooked honey

fructose, fruit juice concentrate, high-fructose corn syrup

aspartame (NutraSweet), sucralose (Splenda), acesulfame potassium

KRYPTONITE

Download your color copy at www.bulletproof.com/diet-roadmap-poster

SUGARS AND SWEETENERS

When it comes to sweetening agents, sugar alcohols like xylitol and erythritol are far and away the most Bulletproof options. Just remember that your xylitol needs to be derived from North American birch wood. If it doesn't say that on the label, chances are good it's made from GMO corn from China. Those two options—xylitol from North American birch wood and erythritol, as well as stevia—are the cleanest and highest on the Bulletproof spectrum. Other things in the top zone are sugar alcohols such as sorbitol and raw honey. Non-GMO dextrose is okay as well. I like raw honey as a sleep hack, too. We seem to understand anecdotally that a teaspoon or a tablespoon will help you sleep better. It must be because it's full of nutrients that help the brain do what it needs to do overnight. That wouldn't likely be true of any cooked or pasteurized honey, though. Steer clear of anything that comes in a little plastic bear.

Options like maple syrup and agave are in the middle zone. They're not the best, but they're not the worst either. Under no circumstances should you eat bottom zone options like aspartame or other sweeteners made in a lab. And, of course, you should absolutely say no to white sugar and high-fructose corn syrup.

BULLETPROOF TIPS AND TECHNIQUES

Now we're just about ready to go. With all that background information, you're ready to start applying what you've learned and working your way to an optimal state of health and performance. Much of the Bulletproof Diet is about the food itself, but it's equally about the ways you should prepare that food.

This cookbook is going to teach you how to use safe, delicious cooking techniques to prepare meals that taste amazing, but also fuel your body and mind to levels of performance beyond what you probably believe you're capable of. We focus on three main types of cooking—gentle baking, blanching and steaming, and sous-vide—because they are the most versatile, flavorful, simple ways to create Bulletproof food. Bulletproof food aims to prevent toxins created by cooking. These small details can make all the difference in your health. They did for me.

When it comes to preparing your food, the worst possible case from a Bulletproof perspective is that you'll burn it. Burning or charring food creates carcinogenic compounds that are linked to cancer. Whatever you do, don't eat foods that have a charred coating! And beyond just avoiding burnt foods, you're also aiming to cook everything as lightly as possible. The foods that work best for the Bulletproof diet have a beautiful composition of fats, and if you heat them up too quickly or to too high a temperature, you change those compounds and ruin the fats. The good news is that there are plenty of easy ways to heat and cook food that tastes great and preserves natural nutrients.

TECHNIQUES

GENTLE BAKING

We talked about this a bit in the healthy fats section (page 20), but whether it's beef, lamb, fish, or chicken, the goal is always to cook meat just enough. Baking at a moderate temperature like 325°F is often just fine. You don't need to sear meat to a sizzle. When you do, you're ruining all the good things about it and destroying its healthful properties. I recommend using a meat thermometer to ensure your meat is done, especially for pork and chicken, whereas beef and lamb are fine medium or medium-rare.

BLANCHING AND STEAMING

Using water is a wonderful way to achieve tender, delicate textures without ruining the composition of your vegetables. Plus, it's fast and easy. For steaming, just place your Bulletproof veggies, like asparagus, broccoli, or cauliflower, in a bamboo steamer or mesh strainer over some simmering water and cover. The veggies will start to soften and tenderize.

For blanching veggies—my favorite way to cook them—you give them a flash-bath in just boiled water. This is great for carrots and harder textured vegetables that need to be softened up. The great benefit to blanching is that by submerging your veggies in boiling water, turning it down, and letting them rest there for a short while (usually under a minute or just a couple minutes), when you drain the water it will take with it some of the harmful substances that some vegetables harbor. This method leaves you with fresh, delicate, nutritionally rich edibles.

Conversely, when you sauté something like spinach or kale, you're cooking them in the toxins that naturally are present, and losing the opportunity to wash them away by cooking in water. By blanching, and to some degree with steaming, you can get rid of any unwanted impurities and enjoy an equally tender, flavorful outcome. That's not possible with sautéing, because any impurities remain on your ingredients.

SOUS-VIDE

I love talking about sous-vide cooking, because this is one of the places where the Bulletproof and the "foodie" approaches to preparing food intersect. While many fancy foodies insist on searing meat, which of course I don't advocate, we can all agree on the wonders of cooking things using the sous-vide method. *Sous-vide* is French for "under vacuum." The method consists of sealing food (usually in airtight plastic bags) and cooking the items in their own (or added) juices or water. Often, one will cook things sous-vide exceedingly slowly, sometimes for days. The goal is to cook everything gently and evenly, and the process produces the most delectable, delicate textures and flavors. It's like whoever invented sous-vide cooking was secretly a Bulletproof eater, because the whole idea is to cook the item through while retaining precious moisture and not overcooking the exterior of the food. Thank you, sous-vide innovator.

WHAT NOT TO DO: MICROWAVE

The other big no-no, besides charring food, is using a microwave. While microwaves are legal and commonly used in the United States, many countries ban them. Microwaves use radiation, which in 2011 the World Health Organization suggested was a class 2B cancer-causing carcinogen. Just don't do it.

EQUIPMENT

When it comes to outfitting your kitchen for Bulletproof living, you don't need to add or change much. You'll want a decent, functioning oven, preferably with a convection setting, but you can also do plenty of prep on the stovetop, be it electric or gas. Natural gas or propane appliances release combustion byproducts into the air that some studies have found are less than optimal. However, electric stoves do have a substantial EMF field that also might be unhealthy. Induction ovens have the strongest EMF field, on par with what leaks out of microwaves. You can even work with a tabletop halogen cooker, which is space-efficient and convenient like a microwave, but without the traumatic cooking process that kills all the nutrients. These cookers are better able to heat things evenly and on all sides, so you get a safe, thorough cooking process.

COOKWARE

The best possible choices for Bulletproof food prep materials are glass, enamel, or ceramic because they don't contain any dangerous metals. Ceramic cookware is ideal because, unlike glass, it can resist cracking in fast temperature changes. The best quality ceramic cookware can be heated to over 2,000°F without cracking. Plus, it has a relatively nonstick surface, it won't scratch, and it's pretty lightweight. That said, ceramic vessels can break if handled roughly or stacked. You can't bang them around like you would with pots and pans.

I recognize that you won't always be baking. Glass and ceramic vessels are optimal when you're gently baking or cooking something in a sous-vide style or bain-marie (a water bath technique that produces a similar effect). Sometimes, you'll want to choose cookware that can also go on the stovetop, at which time I recommend choosing cookware in this order: enamel-coated cast iron (like the popular French brand, Le Creuset), stainless steel, regular cast iron, nonstick.

So those are listed in order from best to worst. If I'm really honest about it, nonstick shouldn't even be on the list because those nonstick coatings always break down and get into the food, tainting it with carcinogenic matter. And for heaven's sake, don't ever use a nonstick-coated pot or pan that is scratched up. In this case, the coating is absolutely loose and will end up in your food. Unless you're trying to give yourself cancer, please don't eat a known carcinogenic substance.

In addition, nonstick-coated pans contain fluoride compounds. So when high heat is applied to the pans, these fluoride compounds and other harmful chemicals in the nonstick coatings can leach into your food. This also happens with aluminum cookware. When this cookware is heated, harmful metallic aluminum ions leach into your food, which has been proven to cause health problems. Stainless steel and cast iron are pretty safe, but high heat still releases the metal ions into food.

DETOX YOUR KITCHEN

Part of Bulletproofing yourself means doing everything you can to reduce the toxicity you take in. Obviously, a big part of that effort means evaluating what you put in your body, be it food, alcohol, or medications. But toxins also live in our environment and degrade our performance simply by being absorbed through our skin or even entering the olfactory system. If you're serious about biohacking your way to Bulletproof living, you'll also want to give your kitchen a thorough going-over.

Start with that seemingly harmless hand soap—and the dishwashing detergent by its side. Standard kitchen cleaning products (especially the ones under the sink) are often chock-full of chemicals that toxify the system. And on a less serious—but still meaningful—note, these same cleansers can change your olfactory sense, which helps you gauge the natural fragrance and taste of your food. When you're eating Bulletproof foods, you want to enjoy all the natural flavor that comes from foods in their purest state. Having cleaning products around can taint your experience—as well as your system. There's

even evidence to show that cleansers can disrupt your endocrine system. Definitely not a recipe for Bulletproofing your body.

Artificial fragrances might seem harmless, or simply annoying, but those perfumes and faux fruit flavors are really noxious compounds. These fragrances, which have nothing to do with nature, are laden with toxic chemical substances that do damage when inhaled or ingested, or if they make contact with your skin. This is true no matter how safe a label may claim the product to be. Artificial fragrances can do great harm even when the concentration is low because the effects are cumulative, and these toxins can get stuck in our cells, compounding the damage over time.

The reason these fragrances are so harmful is that they contain molecules called phthalates. Phthalates, like oily substances, are hard to break down, which is why so many commercial fragrances hang in the air for such an extended period of time. That unnatural smell lingers because it's just hanging there, like toxic sludge in your environment. Guess what—it doesn't break down any more quickly when it's inhaled into your lungs or absorbed into your skin. Just think about that clogging muck the next time you smell something described as "Ocean Breeze" or "Rose Garden." The good news is that avoiding all this nastiness is easy: Just use fragrance-free products and continue on your path to a better, more Bulletproof you.

THE NEXT KITCHEN KILLER: PLASTIC

Plastic is a serious source of toxins in the kitchen. Whether it's dishware, storage containers, drawer liners, and even disposable products like Styrofoam—get rid of it. Plastic, Styrofoam, and resin coatings are made from petroleum products that can leach into your food and drinks. Another common ingredient in these awful products is bisphenol A or BPA for short. BPA is found in a shocking number of our everyday products, from toilet paper to the liners inside metal cans.

BPA is a synthetic hormone, and one that was found, in the '70s and '80s, to cause organ failure and leukemia with toxic levels of exposure. At the same time, those effects weren't evident with lower levels of exposure, but since then we've learned that even in trace amounts, BPAs are harmful. BPAs are nasty any way you slice it, but they are especially evil when heated up, like when you microwave leftovers in a plastic storage container. Never, ever put anything plastic in a microwave (for that matter, try to avoid the microwave altogether, for reasons we've already discussed). When you heat some-

thing up quickly, especially from a very cold state (think about taking out your lunch from the company fridge and popping it in the microwave), it's the best way to give yourself a big serving of BPA for lunch. This is because rapid heating tends to cause more damage to the plastic from heat expansion. Sorry that's not appetizing, but being Bulletproof is about being your best self. And if you're ingesting BPA every day, that's not even close to possible.

If you want to avoid—or minimize—BPA in your kitchen, and your body, remember these rules:

- Avoid water bottled in plastic (glass is OK). Although you may store your bottled water in the fridge, it probably traveled across the blazing hot heartland, in the back of a flatbed truck, getting good and toasty, and the plastic leaching lots of BPA into that "fresh spring" water.
- Instead of drinking bottled water at all, get a good filter for your sink. It will pay for itself within a few months of stopping the frequent purchase of bottled products that only create more landfill anyway.
- Avoid canned foods and drinks whenever possible. There's often a plastic epoxy resin liner inside the metal can.
- Don't microwave food in plastic containers or bags. Don't microwave at

all if you can help it. The toaster oven is a way less-toxic option for reheating.

- Use glass and ceramic dishes for dining, glassware for storage, and stainless steel or wooden utensils.

EATING BULLETPROOF ON THE ROAD

You've probably surmised by now that eating Bulletproof at home is easy. In many ways, it's easier than what I would refer to as a "regular" diet. The challenge for many Bulletproof eaters, myself included, is keeping true to the plan while you're on the road. If you're an executive, salesperson, musician, actor, or other frequent traveler, chances are you're living out of hotel rooms and eating in less-than-optimal places. While this can present some challenges, it's a good opportunity to get creative, and you'll find that there are plenty of ways to get what you need with a few workarounds I've perfected.

HOTEL HACKS

Hotels are tough. Unless you're staying in a 5-star property, with round-the-clock room service and a nothing's-off-limits service approach, you're probably going to have a hard time getting what you need, when you need it. Don't even bother with the mini-bar. The "food" they stock there is nothing short

of a travesty if you're trying to go Bulletproof. When you're living out of a suitcase, you must remember that eggs are your best friend. Whether it's a sad hotel kitchen or the lone convenience store on an otherwise-desolate stretch of highway, chances are you can always find an egg. I buy cartons of them, keep them in the hotel room mini-fridge, and then cook them—are you ready for this?—in the hotel coffee pot. It's actually a rather ingenious little method, and one to make any scoutmaster proud. Just crack your eggs and whisk them with a fork into the pot, and then proceed to scramble them there. I will say that hotels don't love this use of their coffee pots, so I make an effort to clean the pot thoroughly after I'm through.

The next hotel hack, and one that may make you chuckle, is one that was born of a recent attempt to reheat dinner. After assessing the coffee pot and deciding it wasn't the best way to achieve the desired effect, I located the iron. My leftovers were wrapped in aluminum foil, which I smoothed out and used as a wrapper and heat conductor, ironing the remains of my dinner to warm, comforting perfection. I'm sure some of you are scratching your heads about the idea of using aluminum in this hack, but if your food is making contact for such a short period of time, it's not likely to do any damage, first of all. Secondly, when you're on the road, you make sacrifices. You choose the lesser of two evils.

STAYING BULLETPROOF IN RESTAURANTS

Restaurants aren't always Bulletproof-friendly, but you can generally find what you need if you choose the right venue. Obviously, if you're at a nice restaurant, you can almost always get a side of steamed veggies and add butter. If they have grass-fed beef, dig in, and get a nice marbled cut that delivers all those great fats. If the beef isn't grass-fed, go with the leanest cut possible so you're not ingesting the toxins stored in the fat of that meat. You can also generally find a piece of salmon or fish that will do nicely, especially if it's wild-caught. If you're not able to choose an upscale place, and you're left with fast casual places, look for a chain that uses decent ingredients. In some places, you might find a Chipotle, which is a Mexican-themed chain, but one that makes a point to use fresh produce—organic when possible, and, most important, grass-fed beef. If there's nothing

of that caliber around, you shouldn't sweat it. Having a burger or even a slice of pizza once in a blue moon isn't going to kill you (though you may feel a bit sluggish and foggy afterward). Just try to add more veggies and fewer grains whenever possible.

On rare occasions, you may locate a restaurant that is a Bulletproof dream. If you happen to find yourself in the East Bay, just over the bridge from San Francisco, check out my friends' cafe, Mission: Heirloom. Everything they do is right in line with the Bulletproof philosophy and it's delicious to boot. Here, you'll find chefs who cook farm-fresh meat and wild-caught fish just right and minimally prepare vegetables so they retain all their goodness. A few years ago, one could only find food this pure and clean at vegan restaurants, not a place that served all the food groups.

The next chapters share a wealth of the recipes that will allow you to make delicious, optimally designed meals for your best, most powerful self every day of the year as well as on special occasions.

CHAPTER 4

ALL ABOUT THE RECIPES

Now that we've covered all the Bulletproof basics, techniques, and tips, let's get into the actual food you'll be eating. The first thing I'll say is, you're going to love it. These recipes were developed to deliver the ultimate Bulletproof benefits—that was the number one goal—but they were also developed to be delicious and satisfying. You may be surprised to find out that recipes designed to make you perform your best can actually be elegant, impressive, and innovative. I think some people are curious about trying the Bulletproof Diet, but they worry that they'll be bored or be relegated to eating bland, unsatisfying food. Those people will be blown away by these recipes. I don't believe that this approach to eating should set you apart, where you're the one at the party wearing an "I'm on a diet" sandwich board or being "difficult" at a restaurant. In fact, you can have everything you love, from curries to clafoutis.

Once you get familiar with Bulletproof ingredients and techniques, you'll find them flexible and versatile enough to adapt to whatever kinds of dishes you crave. These recipes include everything from comforting classics to multiethnic dishes, all prepared using pure, whole ingredients that help bio-hack your way to becoming Bulletproof. And I'm going to go on the record and challenge any chef to tell me these aren't restaurant-quality delicious. These would fit perfectly on any haute cuisine menu, as the ingredients are fresh and interesting and the preparations are right in step with today's food trends and innovations.

WHOLE FOODS ALL THE WAY

The overarching theme to all these recipes is the quality of the pure, whole ingredients. Food delivers its Bulletproof best when it retains all the nutrients and compounds found in its natural state, so these recipes respect each ingredient and treat them gently, to bring out the inherent flavors and deliver maximum benefit for optimal performance and better brainpower. Each ingredient used has exceptional potential to give you energy and clarity. Everything you'll find here has been reliably sourced for freshness, and nothing's been processed at any stage. I really respect the integrity of the ingredient

and its farm source. It's a standard I set for myself and one you should adopt when you're shopping, too.

My mantra is buy it organic, buy it local, buy it fresh. In that order. I also don't use anything frozen, only whole ingredients bought fresh. The same goes for prepared or prepackaged food—you won't find any of that here. Foods that are packaged or treated have a longer life before you purchase them, which means a likely mold presence or depletion of precious nutrients. You should assume that anything that's been processed or handled in some way to make your life more convenient is robbing you of something essential that the food could otherwise provide. What you gain in ease, you lose in benefit.

With that in mind, every recipe you'll find here meets my Bulletproof standards for high-performance foods and my personal standards for "has to taste great." There are innumerable benefits to cooking and prepping food this way, but one that shouldn't be overlooked is that it makes you a better cook. Going to a farmers' market or quality grocer and carefully selecting your produce, then cooking it with full attention to its properties and essential flavor brings a nuance to the process that naturally makes you more attuned to the culinary process. So the benefits to cooking this way are for mind, body . . . and skill set.

The recipes are broken into main

courses, which are mainly proteins with vegetable sides (although I included a few vegetable mains for when you're protein fasting); sides, which are generally vegetables; soups; smoothies and lattes; and desserts.

While I am a big advocate of using MCT oil in Bulletproof Coffee, I favor natural fats like butter, ghee, marrow, and animal fat for general cooking as they're more versatile and, of course, they impart rich flavor. When it comes to oil, I use Bulletproof Brain Octane or ghee almost everywhere one might have (unwisely) used olive oil. Brain Octane works well for cooking—it has a mild taste that won't overpower any of the flavor the way coconut oil does, so I rub it all over meat, fish, and veggies before cooking them, especially if I'm going for a gentle grilling technique. Always oil the protein, never the heat source. This creates a sealant barrier, much more so than just oiling a pan. I never use high heat with the oil, and I certainly never bring it to smoking. There's just no reason to cook that way, and I've come to view meat that's been handled like that as sort of violently traumatized. Be gentle, people.

Brain Octane is very thin, however—thinner than grapeseed oil—so sometimes I cut it by half with olive oil when I'm not going to cook with it, which is a great way to add a little texture and taste profile while still getting the incredible Bulletproof benefits. You'll also notice I never use more than a tablespoon or two at a time. This is mainly because it's not necessary, but also because taken in larger amounts, Brain Octane oil can require some acclimating for your body. It can be mildly upsetting to the digestive system if you're not accustomed to it; but, as I say, that should never be an issue as I always used it sparingly, just enough to impart the incredible benefits for body and brain.

For proteins, I used a lot of fish from the roadmap selections, as well as grass-fed beef, lamb, eggs, and just a little bit of pastured pork. I generally steer clear of chicken and turkey since it's really difficult to get properly pastured poultry and its nutrient offering is less than optimal. You will find one chicken and one turkey recipe as a concession to those of you who just love the birds. Eating some properly raised poultry every once in awhile won't hurt you; it just doesn't deliver maximum benefit when you're eating to biohack your body.

The vegetable sides heavily favor my favorite Bulletproof foods, like winter squash, leafy greens, and cruciferous vegetables like cabbage. And you'll notice that when it comes to vegetables, I go to town with butter. There's really no better vehicle for all the amazing health benefits of butter than gently steamed or blanched veggies. To bring out the natural flavor of vegetables, I like to use ghee in the beginning of a sauté and then add butter at the end to keep its compounds intact. One of my favorite recipes is a gently steamed kohlrabi with melted butter that just enrobes the vegetable at the end, which tastes amazing, but also keeps the butter as close to whole while giving the dish an elegant finish. This is the opposite of how many chefs approach butter, which is to brown it in the pan before adding vegetables. I don't think that's necessary for great taste, and it definitely doesn't deliver any Bulletproof benefits. You won't find any brown butter here. And you won't miss it.

I use Bulletproof spices whenever possible, not only because they make food taste great, but also because they impart incredible benefits, from antioxidant power to anti-inflammatory action. I'll talk more about their properties in the sidebars of this section as we get deeper into it. For salt, I always use the large grind of coarse sea salt—especially French grey coarse sea salt—nothing kosher and nothing iodized. You should note too that some people treat these kinds of salt just for finishing foods, and they cook with a smaller grind, lesser grade salt. I cooked everything with this coarse grind. It tastes better, it uses less and it's better for you. Bulletproof all the way.

I don't use black pepper because it's nearly impossible to know the quality of the stuff unless you source and grind it yourself.

I do, however, use oregano, which imparts a deep earthy flavor that makes a great pepper substitute.

I'm not a huge fan of cayenne or nuts, but I make concessions where they can be used, if fresh. You'll see the notes about when and how to use them within the particular recipes.

TECHNIQUES

At first glance, you might assume that becoming Bulletproof really limits the way you can prepare foods, but that's not really the case. I think you'll be pleasantly surprised by just how many cooking and preparation techniques—from the everyday to the epicurean—lend themselves to Bulletproof-approved dishes. I blanch, braise, steam, bake, butter-poach, and even (lightly) grill. I use parchment packets, sous-vide techniques, and raw preparations like crudo, ceviche, and carpaccio. I also make comfort classics like chili and stews. Even the most fanatical foodie is not going to be disappointed.

Really, there are very few cooking styles I don't touch upon—except a harsh searing treatment or super high temperatures. You can do so much with these gentler techniques and I find most of them to be right in line with some of the most elevated food concepts out there. We're moving away from old-school cooking with heavy sauces and overly done meats. More and more chefs today are elevating the simple properties of the quality ingredients, making the exercise more about bringing out the essence of the food, rather than burying it. And if you think about it, that really aligns with the Bulletproof philosophy as well: You're bringing out the best of yourself when you go Bulletproof. All the potential and "flavor," if you will, is already there, and you can either bring it out or squelch it. We're treating this food the same way you're going to be treating your body: with utmost respect for its perfect natural potential at its peak.

As always, I used the gentlest cooking methods possible. Slow and low is a great way to approach almost any preparation. Even when I use a grill in these recipes (which is only a couple times), I oil the protein and vegetables liberally, using primarily low flame, and only going to a medium level to get the faintest golden grill marks. You'll be amazed how much "grilled flavor" that imparts. You really don't need to go any higher than that for the same taste experience.

A tip that comes in handy for grilling fish is to cook it skin side down. This really gets you the best possible results. It's a foolproof method that protects the flesh from getting singed if you accidentally go too high

with the flame. I find that until you really know your grill, it's easy to char something depending on where the hotspots are. With fish (and salmon in particular), you can cook it skin side down and still retain all the great omega-3s. Best of all, salmon is optimal served medium-rare, really pink in the middle, so you don't need to worry about it being cooked through. Of course, I love salmon raw and cold-smoked, too, but if you're going for a finished dish, it's hard to beat this for elegance and Bulletproof benefits.

For cookware, I use primarily glass and ceramic. Any time I line a baking sheet to bake something in the oven, I use unbleached parchment paper instead of aluminum foil. I'll make the occasional exception for special dishes that have a specific heating or tenting requirement, but otherwise, there's no reason you can't use unbleached parchment in most cases.

INNOVATION

Obviously biohacking is really an innovative approach to changing your body and mind. It borrows from high-tech, which is, by definition, always innovating. I like to think of these recipes as innovative in their own right. Not only do I use a wide variety of cooking techniques, but I tried to think about surprising combinations of ingredients or unexpected ways to prepare a particular ingredient. Take radishes. Most often, they find their way into salads, which is fine, but it's really not a full expression of their flavor and potential as a focal ingredient. More often than not, they're treated as a sort of peripheral afterthought, like: "There are some radishes I need to use; guess I'll throw them in the salad." The thing is, you braise radishes and suddenly they become this incredible side dish with unexpected complexity; and of course they're amazing paired with butter and some high-grade coarse sea salt. You'll find that recipe on page 115.

You'll also find a cauliflower "couscous" (page 117) which, of course, I put in quotes because it's not the actual Moroccan grain we're talking about. It's become very common for chefs to engage in this kind of wordplay on their menus, calling a portobello mushroom a "steak," or a layered composition of vegetables a "lasagna." Sometimes those descriptions can be disappointing because the result actually tastes nothing like the suggestion and it's really just about being clever, but I like my "couscous" because the steamed cauliflower sautéed with butter really does mimic the texture and taste of a delicate couscous.

I also played around with artichokes. This is also a good time to point out that while fresh artichokes are a little labor-intensive (and really, by that I mean, very little), they are so rewarding in texture and flavor. Plus, the leaves make a great vehicle for dips and proteins like smoked salmon. Besides, canned artichoke is not a Bulletproof-approved food. There's likely a plastic liner filled with BPA in that can, and the product you dump out will be a sad approximation of its former self. Take a few minutes to cut the spikes off a fresh artichoke, shave the stalk, and scoop out the thistly choke. It's so worth it.

I recommend trying to bring a spirit of innovation to these recipes—and to food prep in general. Sometimes the best discoveries come from experimenting and letting things happen.

MAKE THE MOST OF WHATEVER YOU DO

Besides being inherently innovative, the Bulletproof approach is about making the most of every effort. You want everything you eat to provide the maximum benefit for brain and body power. Similarly, with these recipes, you're going to get the most out of every preparation. I've specifically designed these dishes to work hard so you can save leftovers that make a great lunch or lend themselves to another dish you're making later. I like the idea of repurposing and being mindful to not waste *anything*, from your Bulletproof potential to leftover salmon.

Some of the shortcuts and repurposing tricks I've built in include using any leftover salmon baked in parchment for rillettes the next day (which can then get served with crudités at a party *and* go into a lunch for the office the next day). I save any leftover creamed spinach to mix into my creamy guacamole, which can be a party dip, a welcome dollop on a protein-based entrée, or a kid-friendly snack. And after I make and enjoy the duck confit, I roll up leftovers in a cabbage leaf like a spring roll. I love getting the most mileage out of my meals, just like I get the most mileage out of my body when I'm biohacking.

This idea comes into play with sauces, relishes, and dressings, too. I try to make combinations that are versatile and interchangeable. Take my Cilantro-Lime Compound Butter (page 201): Though I use it for bok choy, it would be great on any number of things, including a steak. Salsa verde and tapenade are endlessly delicious and have endless applications. So again, it may take a little time and energy to make these things, but once you have them, you can stretch them, sometimes throughout a week. And that way, you know you're eating delicious, Bulletproof-friendly dishes all day, every day—or at least enough to not worry too much about those moments when you divert from course a little.

Cooking this way also makes it easy to keep up with your social life, as a number of these dishes are elegant enough for entertaining and easy enough to serve at a party. If I'm entertaining, I'd bring out deviled eggs, smoked salmon in radicchio leaves, duck confit spring rolls, creamed guacamole, avocado chocolate mousse, and strawberry semifreddo. Tell me people aren't going to be rolling their eyes in ecstasy at these dishes. And they would never suspect they were eating the most powerful foods to supercharge their system. That's actually a great icebreaker at the party. "Did you know you're eating Bulletproof food?"

I approach eating this way as more of a lifestyle than a diet, and once you think of it that way too, there are no limitations to how creative you can be with preparations and uses. It's an extremely efficient way to eat as well as being delicious and pleasing for a crowd.

KIDS

Having kids is no reason to skip eating Bulletproof foods; in fact, it should be an incentive. We serve one meal per evening at my house, and everyone eats (and loves) it. Because they're so versatile, Bulletproof recipes can easily be transformed into kid-friendly dishes. Take the turkey burger. Roll it into smaller balls or patties and voilà!—it's a kid-size meal of meatballs or sliders. Also, most kids like things like deviled eggs and guacamole. Some will even eat lamb kebabs and salmon rillettes. Bulletproof desserts really hit it out of the park where kids are concerned. Coconut crepes are also perennial favorites with little people.

THE CLASSICS

Like kids, we can be habitual eaters who know what we want and don't want to give it up. I designed these Bulletproof recipes to include lots of familiar dishes; I just supercharged them with Bulletproof ingredients. You like salade Niçoise? Great. I made one substituting trout for tuna and sweet potato for yellow potatoes. There are no tomatoes, but there are eggs, olives, and radishes. I have to say, I like it more than the original (no offense to my friends in Nice). Say you love shepherd's pie. Try the hake and salmon cake instead of cod cake and make carrot and sweet potato mash instead of traditional spuds.

COMFORT CRAVINGS

In addition to creating time-tested favorites, I've included some comfort classics for rainy days or nostalgic moments. We all have dishes that just make us feel good because they're warming and familiar. There's no reason you can't enjoy that experience using Bulletproof ingredients and techniques. Check out my recipes for beef chili and comfort sides that include creamed spinach and "not fried" rice.

OFFICE FOODS

I think the biggest challenge for many people is keeping to Bulletproof standards while eating during a busy workday. It's hard to stop and focus on your food, and nearby stores or cafés may offer limited options if you're minding your meals. The temptation is to bring leftovers and microwave them, but as I explained earlier, I'm anti-microwave, which depletes nutrients at best, and may have harmful effects at worst. I'd recommend taking a good look through these recipes to see which ones keep and travel well (there are plenty) and can be enjoyed cold or at room temperature. My own preferences would be the duck spring rolls, the guacamole with vegetable crudités (makes a great snack), the asparagus with soft-boiled egg, and the trout Niçoise salad. All of these can be easily transported and stored in the fridge at work, and then removed about an hour before you want to eat them.

Eating foods at room temperature is far superior to eating them cold when it comes to taste and texture. The cold temperature shocks your taste buds and you miss out on subtle flavors. Also, textures soften and relax at room temperature, something you've surely noticed if you've ever seen a cold wheel of Brie next to one that's melting and oozing around the plate.

This brings up another hint and related tip: A warm plate makes a big difference in how your food tastes. It's not a thing chefs do just for the ooh and ah factor; a warm plate actually releases aromatics in the food that you can smell and taste (think about warm bread coming out of an oven). While I don't advocate microwaving your food, you can microwave a ceramic plate and place lukewarm food on it to have the same effect.

RECIPES ON THE ROAD

While you may not be able to make these recipes when you travel, you can travel with a recipe you made, and that's my Bulletproof Curry Powder (page 202), which is a mix of powdered turmeric, ginger, cinnamon, Bulletproof VanillaMax (the secret ingredient), and salt. (If you don't have VanillaMax, try a little ground vanilla.) This potent curry blend will gussy up any dish (think about those hotel room eggs you learned how to make) and you can literally carry it around in a vial in your pocket (though you may get some questions at the airport).

DATE NIGHT

Have I convinced you yet that Bulletproof eating is versatile and adaptable to whatever kind of food you prefer? Well, one area we haven't touched upon yet is elegant cuisine fit for a special occasion or date night. I happen to think all these recipes are special and delicious, but sometimes you really want to impress or create a romantic mood, and you're looking for something more elevated in style and preparation. And so I present to you, the Bulletproof Date Night menu. Just read this rundown and tell me you couldn't be sitting at a Michelin-starred restaurant, reading the menu. Eating Bulletproof really is this good.

STARTER
Scallops in Swiss Chard Nest
(page 85)

ENTRÉE
Hanger Steak and Herbed Butter
(page 93) on a bed of Rutabaga and
Celery Root Puree (page 116) with
Winter Squash and Sweet Potato
"Risotto" (page 99)

SIDE
Braised Romaine and Endive
(page 134)

DESSERT
Raspberry-Beet Sorbet (page 183)
with Chocolate Mousse (page 190)
and whipped coconut cream (page 181)

CHAPTER 5

MAINS

My approach to creating Bulletproof entrées is the same approach one would use preparing any main dish: I want it to be filling, versatile, and delicious. It goes without saying that it should be a source for everything your body needs to achieve optimal performance. I've included a side or complementary component for many of these dishes, but you can play around with that—feel free to change them up or choose to integrate something from the next chapter of salads and sides if you prefer. You don't have to live or die by these combinations. They are designed with my favorite flavor profiles and textures in mind, but you can substitute your preferences as you like—it won't change the outcome. Once your fridge and pantry are Bulletproof, you have the ingredients, you have the tools, you have the knowledge—you have total freedom.

Likewise, you can sub in different protein sources once you master the techniques I share here. Braising is a wonderfully versatile way to cook low and slow, extracting all the rich fat and collagen content from meats while imparting deep, hearty flavors. I've braised pork belly here (see page 94), but you can feel free to braise short ribs, oxtail, and other meats. Just follow your tried-and-true Bulletproof techniques for buying: local, fresh, organic, and grass-fed.

The same concept is true for switching up preparations. Once you learn to cook Bulletproof, you have a painter's palette to play with. You know how to source food properly and how to prepare it to best effect, so why not have some fun with it?

In terms of the time required to make main dishes, that is up to you. If you're looking for something quick and effective, head straight for the crudo and salmon rillettes. Not everyone thinks of these dishes as main fare, but why not? They're satisfying, they provide all the benefits you need, and they pair well with all kinds of sides to round things out. Prepare some quick crudo and steamed veggies and you're good to go. Being Bulletproof is about staying efficient and agile, so if it means resetting your perceptions about what's for dinner, let's do it. You'll see this come up with my savory and warm smoothies (pages 170 to 173). They're not traditional, but they are addictive, comforting, and delicious.

If you have some time or you're planning to entertain, you can consider the duck confit, the braised lamb, the pork belly stew, or one of the chilis. Although these take a long time to cook, they aren't that intensive on the prep: it's a matter of setting and forgetting. That confit is going to sit in salt and fat overnight. A braise cooks long, low, and slow, but the results are so worth it, and you can do plenty of other things while it cooks.

When I thought about main-course salads, I didn't want to stick to the expected greens and veggies. Some of the salads here are served warm and are really substantial, like the Trout Niçoise (page 69), which is a really hearty meal. It's filling and, like the others, it's big enough for two people, or two meals.

You can also think about making mains by combining a few of the sides, lighter salads, and vegetables in the next chapter—that's an especially useful strategy when you're protein fasting.

SCALLOPS CRUDO

SERVES 2

When I was a kid, I thought scallops were gross. Now I think they're awesome. Unless you live on an island or near the sea, I recommend buying them frozen because old scallops have high histamines. When you buy them frozen, they're actually fresher. This dish makes a light, satisfying lunch, and you can sub in your favorite seasonal vegetables, such as thinly sliced radishes, celery, or fennel. Also, the beets can be roasted a day ahead of time and kept in the fridge.

½ pound yellow beets, trimmed and washed

½ English cucumber (8 ounces), cut into ⅛-inch-thick slices

1 pound dry sea scallops, cut horizontally into ¼-inch-thick discs

1 teaspoon grated lemon zest

1½ tablespoons lemon juice

1 scallion, finely minced

1 tablespoon high-quality olive oil, plus more for drizzling

1 tablespoon Bulletproof Brain Octane oil (or MCT or coconut oil), optional

½ teaspoon coarse sea salt, plus more to taste

Preheat the oven to 320°F.

Place the beets in an 8 x 8-inch, 2-quart baking pan with ¼ inch water (about 1¼ cups). Cover and bake until tender when pierced with a knife, 45 minutes to 1 hour. Drain and transfer the beets to a bowl to cool to room temperature, about 1 hour. Peel the beets and cut into ⅛-inch-thick slices.

Fan the beets and cucumber on 2 plates. Fan the scallops out along the beets.

In a small bowl, stir together the lemon zest, lemon juice, scallion, olive oil, Brain Octane oil (if using), and salt. Divide the dressing between the plates of scallops, beets, and cucumber. Drizzle with additional olive oil and season with salt to taste.

ASPARAGUS WITH SOFT-BOILED EGGS AND HERB VINAIGRETTE

SERVES 2

Using high-quality, pastured eggs changes this dish from something non-descript to a boldly colored, creamy treat rich in micronutrients. Plus, when you soft-boil your eggs, you're protecting all the good fats. A hard-boiled egg is more inflammatory because the prolonged cooking damages the delicate fats. Get your eggs from a good source and you're good to go.

- 4 large pastured eggs

  Sea salt

- 1 bunch asparagus, trimmed and peeled (if stalks are thick and fibrous)

- ½ teaspoon grated lemon zest

- 1 tablespoon fresh lemon juice

- ½ teaspoon Dijon mustard

- 3 tablespoons finely chopped mixed fresh herbs (such as dill, chives, and parsley)

- 2 tablespoons high-quality olive oil

Have a large bowl of ice water ready. Place the eggs in a small pot and add enough cold water to cover by 2 inches. Bring to a boil over high heat. As soon as it boils, remove from the heat, cover, and let stand 4 minutes. Transfer the eggs to the bowl of ice water and let sit until cold; reserve the ice water (add more ice if necessary). Peel and halve the eggs and season with sea salt.

Cook the asparagus in 1 cup of water until just tender, 2 to 3 minutes. Transfer the asparagus to the ice water to cool completely. Drain.

To make the vinaigrette, in a large bowl, combine the lemon zest, lemon juice, mustard, herbs, and olive oil. Season with sea salt to taste. Add the asparagus and toss to combine. Serve the asparagus with the eggs.

GUACAMOLE CRUDITÉS

SERVES 2

If you read the book, you know that I believe guacamole is a superior food group in and of itself. It's a fat that makes you feel good. This nutrient-dense version takes regular guacamole and ramps up the green veggie power. By adding spinach, you make a spinach-dip-meets-guacamole hybrid. Purists, please don't be offended; this creation is something else entirely. And as an extra bonus, you can add bacon, especially if it's baked.

1 cup Coconut Creamed Spinach (page 114), chilled

2 avocados, pitted and peeled

2½ tablespoons fresh lime juice

2 tablespoons chopped fresh cilantro leaves

Sea salt

2½ cups assorted Bulletproof vegetables for dipping: raw radishes, fennel, carrots, celery, or cucumber; steamed broccoli, green beans, parsnip, or sweet potato

In a food processor, puree the creamed spinach. Add the avocado, lime juice, and cilantro and pulse to a thick puree. Season with sea salt to taste. Serve with vegetables for dipping.

DEVILED EGGS WITH ENDIVE AND SALMON

SERVES 2

This makes a great on-the-go packed lunch, filled with good saturated fats. It also doubles as a nice dinner option when paired with a salad and an herb vinaigrette (from Asparagus with Soft Boiled Eggs on page 62). Remember not to overcook the yolk—just enough so it will hold up texturally. This recipe is a way to get your fat and protein in a hurry. Eat a handful and that's your meal.

4   large pastured eggs

¼   cup Bulletproof Mayonnaise (page 205)

1   teaspoon fresh lemon juice

1   teaspoon Bulletproof Curry Powder (page 202)

1   tablespoon finely chopped fresh chives, cilantro, or parsley

   Sea salt

4   ounces smoked salmon, cut into 8 pieces

8   Belgian endive or radicchio leaves, separated

Have a large bowl of ice water ready. Fill a small pot with enough cold water to cover the eggs plus another 2 inches. Cover and bring to a boil over high heat. As soon as it boils, remove from the heat and let stand covered for 9 minutes. Transfer the eggs to the bowl of ice water and let sit until the eggs are cold, about 5 minutes.

Peel and halve eggs, setting the whites aside. Pass the egg yolks through a fine-mesh sieve over a medium bowl. Add the mayonnaise, lemon juice, curry powder, herbs, and sea salt to taste, mixing well. Spoon or pipe the yolk mixture into the egg halves.

Place a piece of smoked salmon atop each endive leaf and top with a deviled egg half.

DUCK SPRING ROLLS

SERVES 2

I love to use this fancy dish to impress people. It takes a little prep, but it tastes amazing. It's the perfect way to turn that Duck Confit (page 98) into an easy-to-eat finger food to pass around at parties.

4	teaspoons apple cider vinegar
	Sea salt
5 or 6	red or green cabbage leaves, center ribs removed
1	cup shredded carrots (about 2)
2	celery stalks, thinly sliced (about $^2/_3$ cup)
2	duck confit legs (page 98), warmed and meat shredded
$^1/_3$	cup cilantro leaves
2 to 3	teaspoons fresh lime juice (to taste)

In a large high-sided skillet with a lid, bring 1 cup water, 1 teaspoon of the vinegar, and 1 teaspoon sea salt to a simmer. Add the cabbage, cover, and steam until tender, about 4 minutes. Remove the cabbage and set aside.

In a bowl, toss together the carrots, celery, duck, cilantro, lime juice, and remaining 3 teaspoons vinegar.

Fill the cabbage leaves with the duck mixture, rolling each up like a spring roll. Serve immediately.

RADICCHIO, ENDIVE, AND PARSNIP SALAD

SERVES 2

Let's be honest, parsnips are an acquired taste. The first time I had them, I was at a steakhouse called Birks in Silicon Valley, where they were pureed and served with the ribeye. I told the chef, Maurice, they weren't as good as creamed spinach. Then I realized they are a great source of nonsugary carbs low in toxins. This salad is perfect to have when you're in maintenance mode and not protein fasting. The walnuts are high in micronutrients and omega-6 oils so they're a great addition as long as they are mold-free and high quality from a reliable source.

1 large parsnip (12 ounces), peeled and cut into 1/2-inch chunks

2 teaspoons grainy mustard

1 teaspoon raw honey (optional)

2 teaspoons fresh lemon juice

1 tablespoon high-quality olive oil

1 tablespoon Bulletproof Brain Octane oil (or MCT or coconut oil)

Sea salt

1 head radicchio (8 ounces), leaves separated and coarsely torn

2 Belgian endives (12 ounces each), halved and cut crosswise into 1/2-inch slices

1/2 cup fresh parsley leaves

1/3 cup walnuts, coarsely chopped (optional)

In a medium saucepan fitted with a steamer insert, bring 2 cups of water to a simmer over medium heat. Add the parsnips, cover, and steam until just tender, about 4 minutes. Set aside to cool slightly.

Meanwhile, in a small bowl, whisk together the mustard, honey (if using), lemon juice, olive oil, and Brain Octane oil. Season with sea salt to taste.

Assemble the radicchio, endives, parsnip, and parsley in a bowl. Drizzle with the mustard vinaigrette. If desired, top with walnuts.

ROMAINE SALAD AND GINGER DRESSING

This is a cool way to achieve taste in a dressing you'd never expect. It has strong flavor, great color, and consistency. The Brain Octane oil carries the flavor of the ginger to your palate and helps you feel fuller faster. It's great on other chopped vegetables, too, such as arugula.

3	carrots (8 ounces), cut into 1-inch pieces
1	piece (1½ inches) fresh ginger
2	tablespoons Bulletproof Brain Octane oil (or MCT or coconut oil)
3	tablespoons high-quality olive oil
2	tablespoons apple cider vinegar
¼	cup water
	Sea salt
1	head romaine lettuce, torn
2	radishes, sliced
1	small zucchini, thinly shaved with a vegetable peeler

In a medium saucepan, bring 1 inch of water to a simmer over medium heat. Add the carrots, cover, and cook until tender, about 8 minutes. Drain and let the carrots cool to room temperature, about 10 minutes.

Transfer the carrots to a food processor or heavy-duty blender. Add the ginger, Brain Octane oil, olive oil, vinegar, and water and process until smooth. Season with sea salt to taste. Chill for about 20 minutes or up to 1 hour before using.

Combine the romaine, radishes, and zucchini in a bowl and toss with the dressing.

SALMON RILLETTES AND ROMAINE

When you eat a lot of sockeye salmon, you often have leftovers. By stirring a few things together, you can achieve amazing flavor, making it more creamy and delicious than it was the first time around. It's a great way to get your omega 3s and saturated fats at once. To be honest, I had to work with chefs to figure out what to call this dish. They steered me toward a fancy French name. I would never have known to call it rillettes, but I'm going to stick with it.

3 tablespoons grass-fed unsalted butter, at room temperature

1 scallion, minced

8 ounces cooked wild salmon (see Perfect Parchment-Baked Salmon, page 77)

3 ounces smoked salmon, finely chopped

4 teaspoons fresh lemon juice

1 tablespoon capers, coarsely chopped, plus more for garnish

2 teaspoons finely chopped fresh tarragon

Sea salt

10 romaine leaves, for serving

In a small bowl, stir together the butter, scallion, cooked salmon, smoked salmon, lemon juice, and capers until combined. Mix in the tarragon and season with sea salt to taste. Scoop into the romaine leaves, garnish with capers, and serve.

TROUT NIÇOISE

SERVES 2

I grew up catching rainbow trout in New Mexico and I still remember how delicious it was. This dish takes me back to that time. You can substitute other seasonal vegetables for the green beans, fennel, and sweet potato, such as asparagus, celery, and celery root. This way you can enjoy smoked trout with fresh flavors year-round.

³/₄ pound green beans

1 sweet potato (8 ounces), peeled, halved lengthwise, and cut crosswise into ¹/₂-inch slices

1 teaspoon grainy mustard

1 tablespoon apple cider vinegar

5 tablespoons high-quality olive oil

Sea salt

1 tablespoon tarragon leaves, coarsely chopped

2 large pastured eggs, hard-boiled, peeled, and halved

4 radishes, thinly sliced

1 small fennel bulb (8 ounces), trimmed, cored, and thinly sliced

¹/₃ cup Kalamata or Niçoise olives, pitted

¹/₂ avocado, pitted, peeled, and sliced

5 ounces smoked trout, flaked

Have a large bowl of ice water ready. In a large pot fitted with steamer insert, bring 2 cups of water to a simmer. Add the green beans, cover, and steam until crisp-tender, 4 to 5 minutes. Transfer the beans to the ice water to stop the cooking.

Add the sweet potatoes to the steamer (add more water if necessary). Cover and steam until tender, 7 to 8 minutes. Set aside to cool.

In a large bowl, whisk together the mustard, vinegar, and olive oil. Season with sea salt to taste and stir in the tarragon.

Assemble the salads with the green beans, sweet potato, eggs, radishes, fennel, olives, avocado, and smoked trout. Dress with the tarragon vinaigrette.

WINTER VEGETABLE SALAD

SERVES 2

This hearty winter salad can be reinvented using a host of seasonal vegetables like celery root, rutabaga, or broccoli. My favorite thing about this dish is the way we reuse the bacon fat to make the flavor explode. You just can't help but smile with this much bacon flavor.

2	slices thick-cut pastured bacon
2½	pounds winter vegetables such as sweet potatoes, carrots, parsnip, winter squash, and turnip, cut into 1-inch pieces
4	teaspoons Bulletproof Brain Octane oil (or MCT or coconut oil)
6	teaspoons high-quality olive oil
1	tablespoon chopped fresh herbs (such as thyme, rosemary, and oregano)
	Sea salt
½	small head cabbage (9 ounces), cored and cut lengthwise into 1-inch-thick slices
2	teaspoons apple cider vinegar
2	tablespoons chopped raw almonds

Preheat the oven to 320°F. Line a baking sheet with parchment paper.

Arrange the bacon on the baking sheet and bake until just cooked through, but not browned, about 10 minutes. Let cool and coarsely chop. Reserve the pan and bacon fat and leave the oven on.

Add the vegetables to the bacon fat in the pan and toss with the Brain Octane oil, 4 teaspoons of the olive oil, the herbs, and salt to taste. Bake until just beginning to soften, about 20 minutes.

Add the cabbage to the baking sheet, tossing to combine, and continue to bake, tossing once, until all vegetables are tender, about 30 minutes. Drizzle the vegetables with the remaining 2 teaspoons olive oil and the vinegar and sprinkle with the bacon and almonds. Serve warm or at room temperature.

GREENS WITH CREAMY DRESSING

SERVES 2

To be perfectly Bulletproof with this recipe, go a bit more soft-cooked on the egg, but if you're not worried about the cholesterol, this recipe works well with hard-cooked eggs. Either way, you'll add a nice protein kick to a peppery arugula salad. You can also use watercress or radicchio—whichever green you prefer.

2 large pastured eggs, hard-boiled, peeled, and halved

2 tablespoons Bulletproof Mayonnaise (page 205)

1 scallion, white part only, finely minced

2 tablespoons fresh lemon juice

2 teaspoons high-quality olive oil

Sea salt

1 head romaine lettuce, coarsely chopped

2 cups arugula leaves (1½ ounces)

¼ cup skin-on sliced almonds (optional)

Chop the egg whites and finely grate the egg yolks.

In a small bowl, whisk together the mayonnaise, scallion, lemon juice, and olive oil. Season the dressing with sea salt to taste.

In a large bowl, toss the romaine, arugula, egg whites, and egg yolks with the dressing. Sprinkle with the almonds (if using) and serve.

BEEF BACON LOAF

SERVES 2, WITH LEFTOVERS

I've never been a big fan of any dish described as a loaf. But this is a new spin on your mom's meat loaf, which avoids breadcrumbs and other fillers, packing in green vegetables and incredible bacon flavor. Pro tip: If you have any bacon fat reserved from the cooking process, you can add it into the loaf.

- 1 bunch scallions, white and light green parts only, thinly sliced
- 2 carrots, finely chopped
- ½ bunch collard greens, ribs removed, leaves finely chopped (optional)
- 2 pounds grass-fed ground beef
- 4 large pastured egg whites

- 1 bunch scallions, greens parts only, finely chopped
- 1 cup chopped cooked pastured bacon
- 1 tablespoon ground cinnamon
- 2 teaspoons ground allspice
- ½ teaspoon ground cloves
- 2 teaspoons coarse sea salt

Preheat the oven to 325°F.

In a medium skillet over low heat, cook the sliced scallions and carrots until just crisp-tender, about 7 minutes. Set aside.

If using collard greens, add them to the same pan and cook until just wilted, about 2 minutes.

In a large bowl, combine cooked scallions, carrots, and collard greens (if using). Add the ground beef, egg whites, scallion greens, bacon, cinnamon, allspice, cloves, and sea salt. Mix well to combine. Form into a loaf and place in a 9 x 5 x 2-inch loaf pan.

Bake until just cooked through, 35 to 40 minutes. Let rest in the pan about 10 minutes before slicing.

EGG WHITE CURRY LOAF

SERVES 2, WITH LEFTOVERS

This recipe works because it's a great way to use the egg whites when you've allocated the yolks for something else, like my Bulletproof "Get Some" Vanilla Ice Cream (page 180). When you've got the leftover egg whites from that recipe, you can use them here. Keep in mind that leeks are a member of the allium family so be mindful of your intake. They're generally okay—less of a red flag than garlic.

1 tablespoon grass-fed unsalted butter or ghee, for the baking pan

1 leek, well washed, white and light green parts only, thinly sliced

1 small fennel bulb, finely chopped

3 celery stalks, finely sliced

1 cup thinly sliced napa cabbage

3 kale leaves, finely chopped

1 medium zucchini, thinly sliced

½ cup water

1 tablespoon grated fresh ginger

6 large pastured egg whites

1 teaspoon dried thyme

1 teaspoon ground cumin

1 teaspoon ground coriander

1 teaspoon ground turmeric

1 teaspoon sea salt

½ cup coconut butter, slightly melted

Preheat the oven to 320°F. Grease a 9 x 5 x 2-inch loaf pan with the butter.

In a Dutch oven or large pot, combine the leek, fennel, celery, napa cabbage, kale, zucchini, and water and cook over medium-low heat, stirring occasionally, until slightly tender, about 10 minutes. Transfer to a large bowl to cool slightly, about 5 minutes.

Add the ginger, egg whites, thyme, cumin, coriander, turmeric, sea salt, and coconut butter to the vegetables. Mix well to combine. Form into a loaf and press the mixture into the buttered pan. Bake until just cooked through and egg is set, about 55 minutes. Let cool in the pan about 15 minutes before slicing.

LAMB CUMIN LOAF

SERVES 2, WITH LEFTOVERS

Here, my Bulletproof lamb gets a Chinese flavor spin with a big cumin kick. A lot of people don't use cumin regularly because it's not well known to them. Where I grew up, in New Mexico, we put cumin in many things, including guacamole. I use it here for a dash of flavor and a touch of nostalgia.

1   leek, well washed, white and light green parts only, thinly sliced

1   head bok choy, stalks only, thinly sliced

3   medium carrots, finely chopped

3   tablespoons water

4   large pastured egg whites

1   pound ground lamb

1   teaspoon apple cider vinegar

1   tablespoon ground cumin

1   teaspoon cumin seeds

2   teaspoons dried oregano

1   teaspoon sea salt

Preheat the oven to 320°F.

In a medium saucepan, combine the leek, bok choy, carrots, and water. Cover and cook over medium-low heat until tender, about 10 minutes. Transfer to a large bowl to cool slightly, about 5 minutes.

Add the egg whites, ground lamb, vinegar, ground cumin, cumin seeds, oregano, and sea salt. Mix well to combine. Form into a loaf and place in a 9 x 5 x 2-inch loaf pan.

Bake until just cooked through, 35 to 40 minutes. Let rest in the pan for 10 minutes before slicing.

SOCKEYE SALMON DILL LOAF

SERVES 2, WITH LEFTOVERS

If you're like me, you don't always have time to make a fancy meal, so when you have leftovers, you find a way to add elements that create a delicious next meal. This dish is just such a solution, in which the dill and coconut breathe new life into your remaining salmon.

- 1 leek, well washed, white and light green parts only, thinly sliced
- 2 cups chopped arugula
- 1 cup chopped fresh flat-leaf parsley leaves
- 2 teaspoons dried dill
- 1 teaspoon sea salt
- 6 large pastured egg whites
- 2 pounds wild sockeye salmon, cooked, chilled, and flaked into small pieces

Preheat the oven to 320°F.

In a small skillet, cook the leek over medium-low heat until fragrant, about 3 minutes. Transfer to a large bowl to cool slightly.

Add the arugula, parsley, dill, salt, and egg whites. Mix well to combine. Carefully fold in the salmon. Form into a loaf and place in a 9 x 5 x 2-inch loaf pan.

Bake until just cooked through and the egg white is set, about 50 minutes. Let cool in the pan slightly before slicing.

BRAISED INDIE SALMON

SERVES 2, WITH LEFTOVERS

Since I became Bulletproof, I don't really ever think about bread and gluten, but I used to love the naan bread from Amber India in Silicon Valley, which you could get spiced with nigella seeds. This is my answer to that cool flavor from India. You can find nigella seeds in Indian markets, where it's often labeled *kalonji*.

1	leek, well washed and thinly sliced (optional)
2	celery stalks, thinly sliced
2	carrots, finely chopped
5	spears baby asparagus, trimmed and finely chopped
1	can (14 ounces) coconut milk, well shaken
1	head bok choy, cored and chopped
4	wild sockeye salmon fillets (3 ounces each)
1/2	teaspoon cumin seeds
1/2	teaspoon fennel seeds
1/2	teaspoon black mustard seeds
1/2	teaspoon fenugreek seeds
1/2	teaspoon nigella seeds
1	teaspoon sea salt
1/2	cup coconut oil
1	tablespoon Bulletproof Brain Octane oil (or MCT or coconut oil)

In a medium pot, combine the leek, celery, carrots, and asparagus and cook, stirring often, until softened, about 4 minutes.

Add the coconut milk, bok choy, salmon, cumin, fennel, mustard seeds, fenugreek, nigella seeds, and sea salt. Cover and simmer until the vegetables are tender and the fish is just cooked through, about 10 minutes.

Plate and drizzle with the coconut oil and Brain Octane oil.

PERFECT PARCHMENT-BAKED SALMON

SERVES 2

Salmon is one of the perfect superfoods if you cook it just right. If you go too long, it's no *bueno*. This recipe takes the guesswork out, so it's a can't-miss way to get your omega-3s. And you can substitute any Bulletproof fish here, just note that the cooking times will vary depending on the fish's thickness. Try pairing this with the Carrot and Cabbage Slaw (page 122) or the Low-Roasted Broccoli Rabe (page 129).

2   center-cut wild salmon fillets (8 ounces each)

1   teaspoon Bulletproof Brain Octane oil (or MCT or coconut oil)

    Sea salt

1   tablespoon grass-fed unsalted butter

1   tablespoon minced fresh herbs (such as chives, parsley, or dill)

    Lemon wedges, for serving

Preheat the oven to 320°F.

Place the salmon on a piece of parchment paper on a baking sheet. Rub the fillets with Brain Octane oil, season with sea salt, and top with the butter. Wrap the parchment around the fish, folding seams and tucking them to ensure steam does not escape.

Bake until fish is medium-rare, about 18 minutes. Sprinkle with the herbs and a squeeze of lemon.

GRILLED SALMON AND ZUCCHINI

SERVES 2

For years, grilling was my go-to method for cooking salmon, but that method can lead to inflammatory foods. The trick is not to char the fish and keep the fat from hitting the hot coals. Cook it gently and lower the flame as needed.

1 pound zucchini, cut into ½-inch slices

2 tablespoons plus 2 teaspoons Bulletproof Brain Octane oil (or MCT or coconut oil)

2 teaspoons minced fresh oregano

4 tablespoons fresh lemon juice

4 teaspoons high-quality olive oil

Sea salt

2 skin-on wild salmon fillets (8 ounces each), skin scored lightly

4 teaspoons finely chopped fresh herbs (such as chive, parsley, or oregano)

Heat a grill pan over (or fire up your grill to) medium-high heat.

In a medium bowl, toss the zucchini with 2 tablespoons of the Brain Octane oil. Grill lightly, in batches, reducing the heat or flame to low and turning halfway, until the zucchini is crisp-tender, 6 to 8 minutes. Set the grill pan aside (or leave the grill on). Sprinkle the zucchini with the oregano, 2 tablespoons of the lemon juice, the olive oil, and sea salt to taste. Set aside.

If using a grill pan, heat over medium-high heat. Rub the salmon with the remaining 2 teaspoons Brain Octane oil and sprinkle with sea salt. Place the salmon on the grill surface, skin-side-down, and cook about 6 minutes, reducing the heat to medium-low as needed to avoid charring the skin. Carefully flip the fillets and cook until fish is medium-rare, about 3 minutes longer.

Top the fish with herbs and the remaining 2 tablespoons lemon juice. Season to taste with sea salt and serve with the zucchini.

CHILLED POACHED SALMON, WATERCRESS SAUCE, AND GREEN BEANS

SERVES 2

This is a simple make-ahead recipe that tastes good thanks to the creaminess from Bulletproof mayonnaise. This dish satisfies and doesn't require lot of work. Also, you can use any leftover watercress sauce as a base for the deviled eggs on page 64.

2 skinless wild salmon fillets (8 ounces each)

1 tablespoon grass-fed unsalted butter

1 bunch watercress

1/3 cup packed fresh basil leaves

1/2 cup Bulletproof Mayonnaise (page 205)

2 1/2 teaspoons fresh lemon juice

Sea salt

8 ounces green beans

1 tablespoon Bulletproof Brain Octane oil (or MCT or coconut oil)

In a medium saucepan, combine the salmon and butter and add enough water to just cover the salmon. Cover the pan, bring to a simmer over medium heat, and simmer until the salmon is just cooked through, about 12 minutes total. Use a fish spatula or slotted spoon to transfer the salmon to a plate. Drain the saucepan and set aside to use again. Refrigerate the salmon until chilled, about 1 hour.

Have a large bowl of ice water ready. Add 1/4 cup tap water to the reserved saucepan. Cover and bring to a simmer over medium heat. Add the watercress, cover, and cook until wilted, about 1 minute. Transfer the watercress to the ice water to stop the cooking. Squeeze out excess water and coarsely chop.

In a blender, combine the watercress, basil, and mayonnaise and process until smooth. Add 1 teaspoon of the lemon juice and season with salt to taste.

Add 1 cup of water to the saucepan, cover, and bring to a simmer over medium heat. Add the green beans, cover, and cook until just tender, 2 to 3 minutes. Drain the beans and toss with the Brain Octane oil, remaining 1 1/2 teaspoons lemon juice, and salt to taste.

Serve the salmon with the watercress sauce and green beans.

HAKE AND SALMON CAKES

SERVES 2 (2 CAKES PER PERSON)

These are ridiculously delicious. The sweetness of the rice flour makes the creamy fish flavor explode. Plus, any leftovers make a great lunch option. You can reheat these cakes, covered, in a 320°F oven for 6 to 8 minutes. Serve with some arugula, avocado slices, Brain Octane oil, and a drizzle of lemon juice or the Carrot and Cabbage Slaw on page 122.

1	large pastured egg
1	tablespoon fresh lemon juice
1	tablespoon Dijon mustard
	Sea salt
2	tablespoons olive oil
1	tablespoon Bulletproof Brain Octane oil (or MCT or coconut oil)
$\frac{1}{2}$	pound skinless wild sockeye salmon, cut into $\frac{1}{4}$-inch cubes
$\frac{1}{2}$	pound skinless hake, cut into $\frac{1}{4}$-inch cubes
$\frac{1}{4}$	cup finely chopped fresh flat-leaf parsley
$\frac{1}{4}$	cup sweet rice flour
2	teaspoons ghee

Line a plate with parchment paper and set aside.

In a food processor, pulse together the egg, lemon juice, mustard, and a pinch of sea salt. As it pulses, drizzle the oils slowly into the food processor to combine. Add half of the salmon and hake and pulse to a coarse paste. Fold in the remaining fish and parsley, then fold in the sweet rice flour. With wet hands, to prevent sticking, divide the mixture into 4 patties 3 inches wide and $\frac{3}{4}$ inch thick. Place the cakes on the plate and refrigerate until chilled and firm, about 1 hour.

Preheat the oven to 320°F.

In a large ovenproof skillet, melt the ghee over medium heat. Add the fish cakes to the pan and cook, turning once, until firm on the outside, about 8 minutes. Transfer the pan to the oven and bake until the cakes are hot, about 10 minutes.

HAKE OR COD IN PARCHMENT WITH SALSA VERDE

SERVES 2

Both hake and cod work well here, but you can use this salsa verde on the Bulletproof fish of your choice. Unlike other salsa verdes, which tend to include tomatillos, this version includes nothing from the nightshade family.

2 hake or cod fillets ($\frac{1}{2}$ pound each)

Sea salt

1 tablespoon grass-fed unsalted butter, cut into small pieces

2 lemon slices ($\frac{1}{4}$ inch thick)

1 fennel bulb (10 ounces), trimmed, cored, and thinly sliced

Salsa Verde (page 203)

Preheat the oven to 320°F. Line a baking dish with parchment paper. Place the fillets on the parchment paper, season with salt, and dot with the butter. Place a lemon slice on each fillet. Wrap the parchment around the fillets, folding seams, and tucking in the sides so no steam escapes. Bake until the fish is just cooked through, 20 to 25 minutes, depending on thickness.

Toss the fennel with 2 tablespoons of the salsa verde. Serve the fennel and remaining salsa with the fillets.

WILD COD, TAPENADE, AND BUTTER-POACHED ASPARAGUS

SERVES 2

Tapenade is one of those things that you might imagine is a luxury, but on a high fat diet, it's its own food group. It's not expensive and easy enough to make. The combo of ghee, oil, and olives in the tapenade complements the fish and makes me feel like I'm eating pizza.

¼	cup ghee or grass-fed unsalted butter
1	bunch asparagus, trimmed and peeled
	Sea salt
1	teaspoon grated lemon zest
2	wild cod fillets (6 to 8 ounces each)
½	teaspoon fresh lemon juice
½	cup Tapenade (page 204)

In a large skillet with a lid, melt the ghee over medium heat. Add the asparagus and cook, covered, turning occasionally, until just tender, 8 to 10 minutes. Transfer the asparagus to a plate, season with sea salt to taste, and toss with the lemon zest.

Return the skillet to the stove and reduce the heat to low. Season the cod with salt to taste and add to the pan. Cook gently, covered, until just cooked through, about 12 minutes.

To serve, drizzle the fish with the lemon juice and serve with the tapenade and asparagus.

ASPARAGUS COOKING TIME: The cooking time for the asparagus will vary with its thickness; thinner spears cook more quickly, while thicker spears take longer.

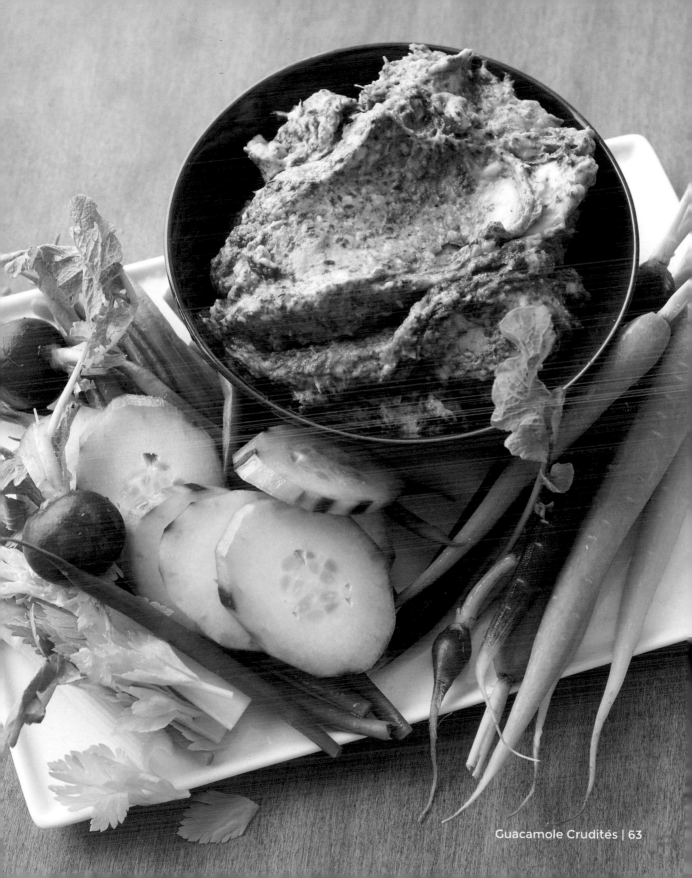

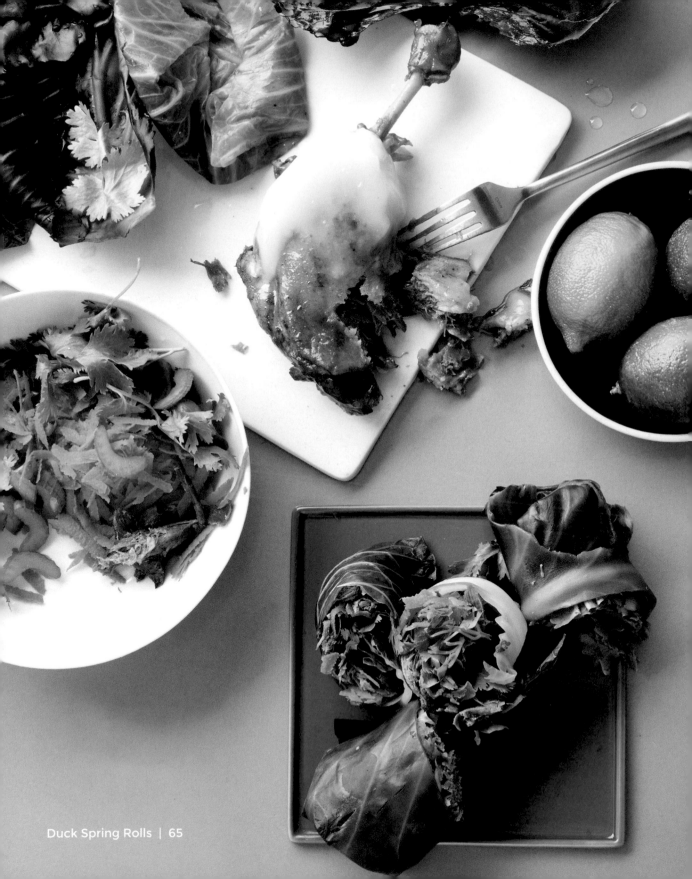

Duck Spring Rolls | 65

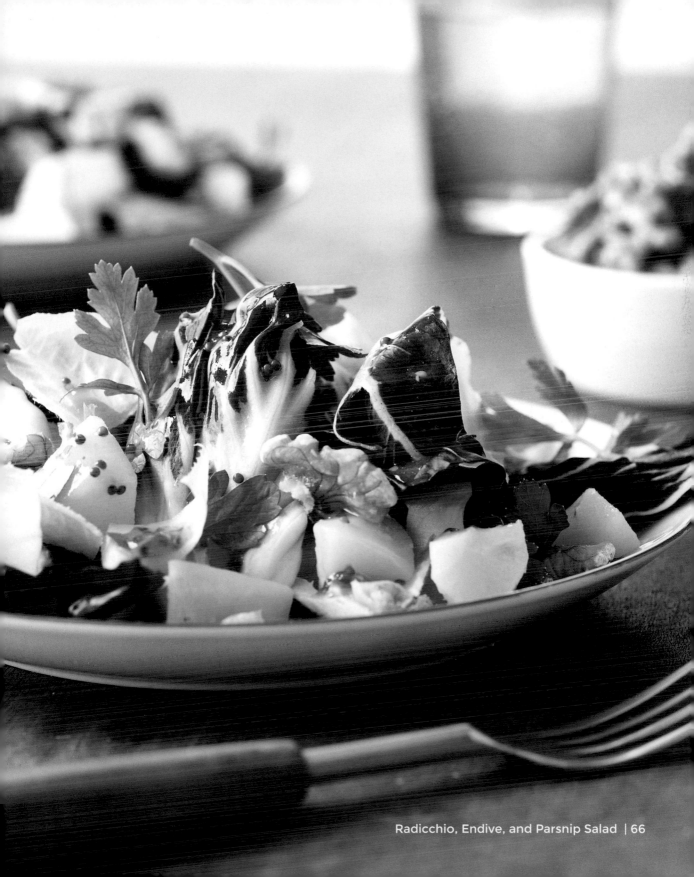

Radicchio, Endive, and Parsnip Salad | 66

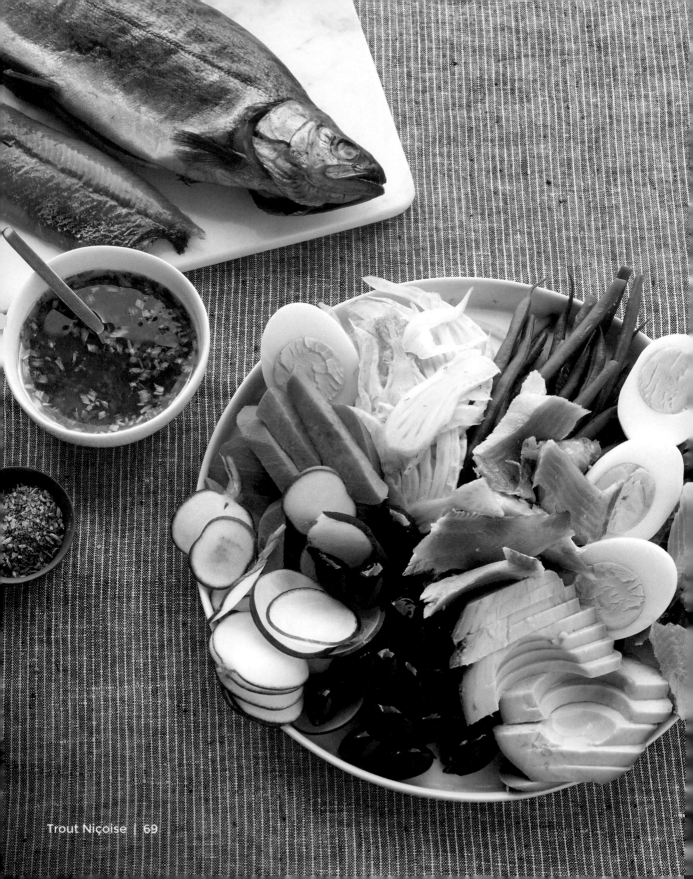

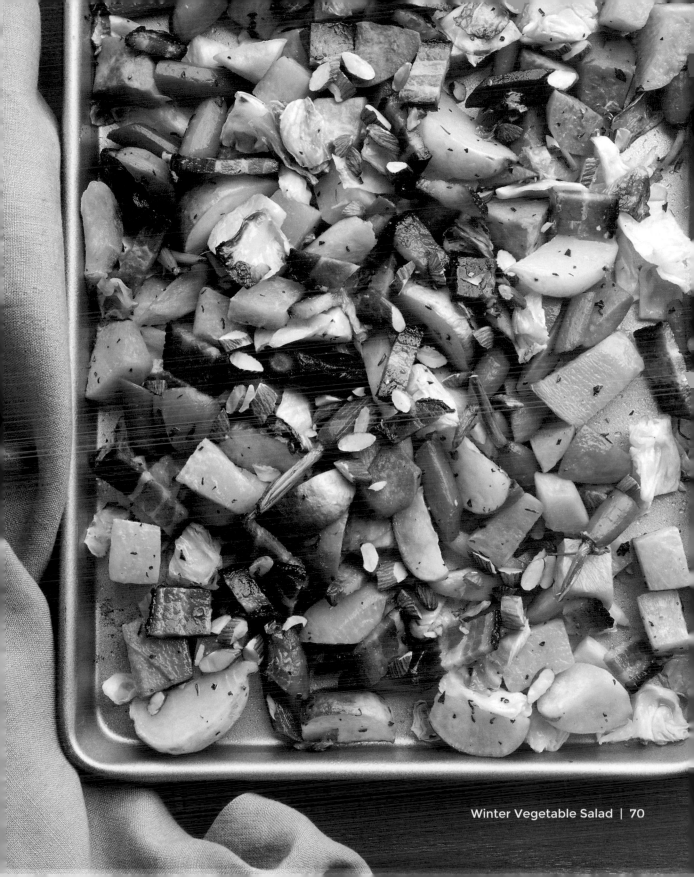

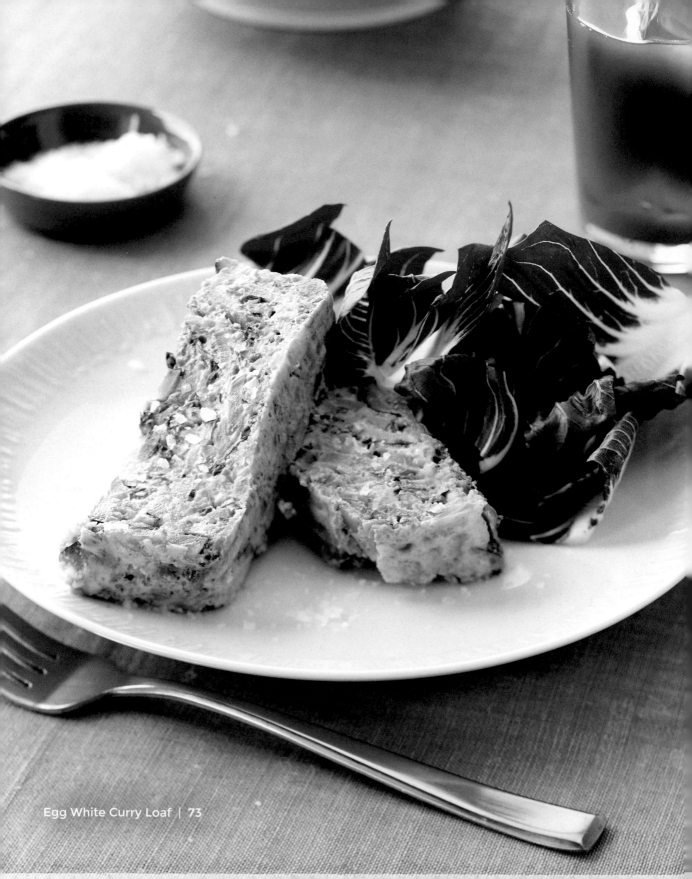

Egg White Curry Loaf | 73

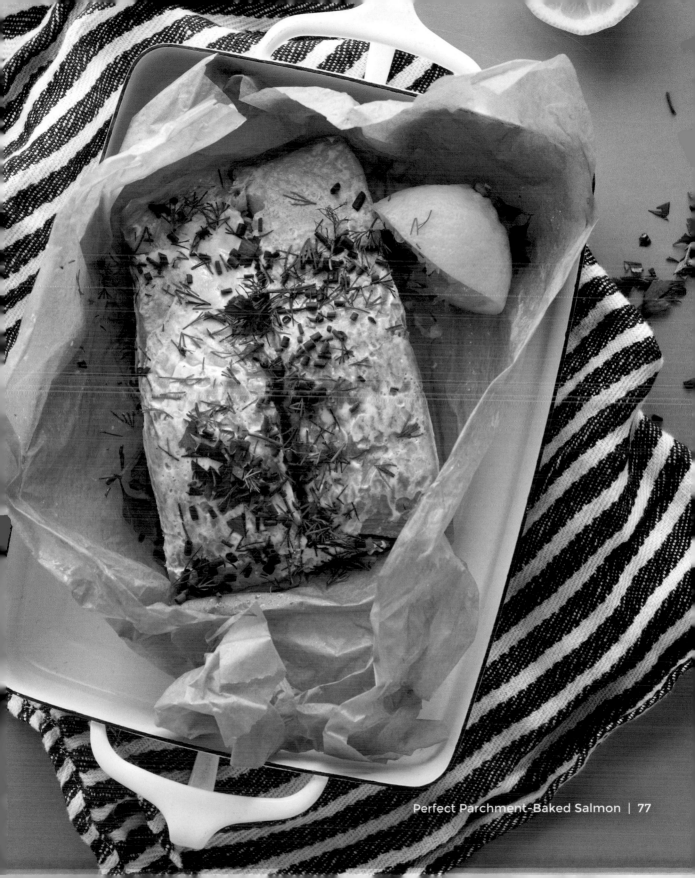

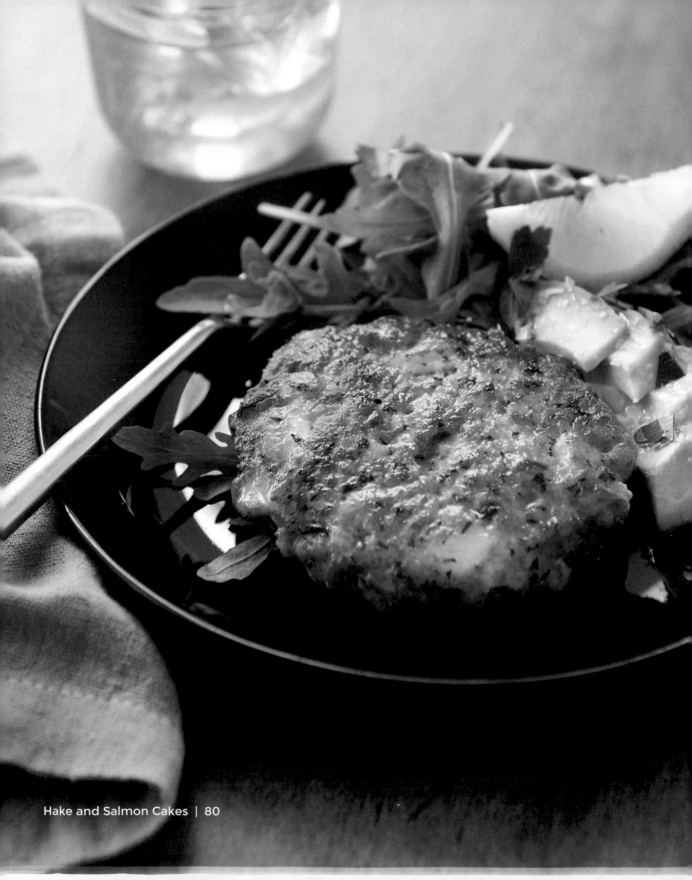

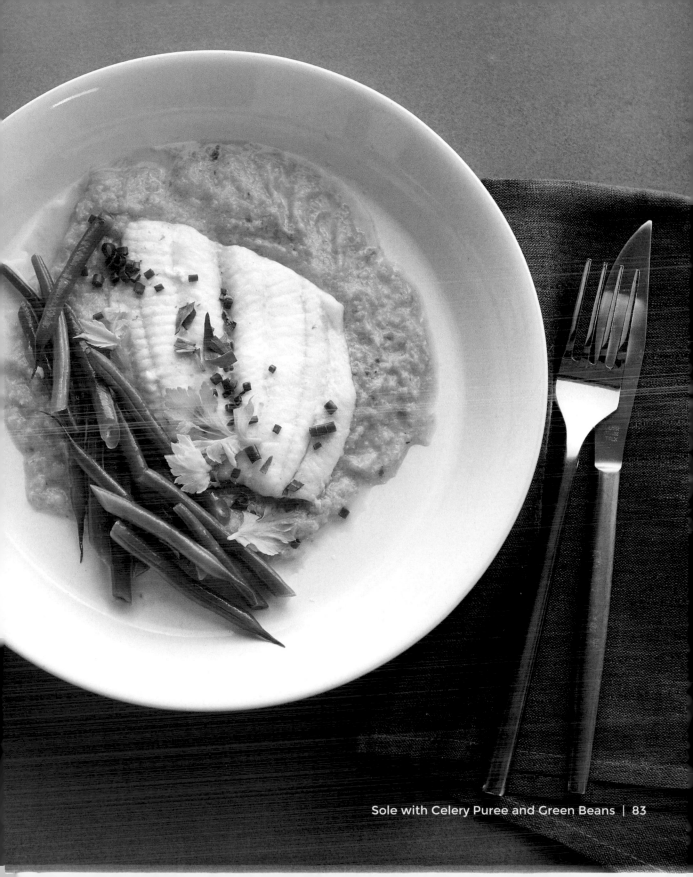

Sole with Celery Puree and Green Beans | 83

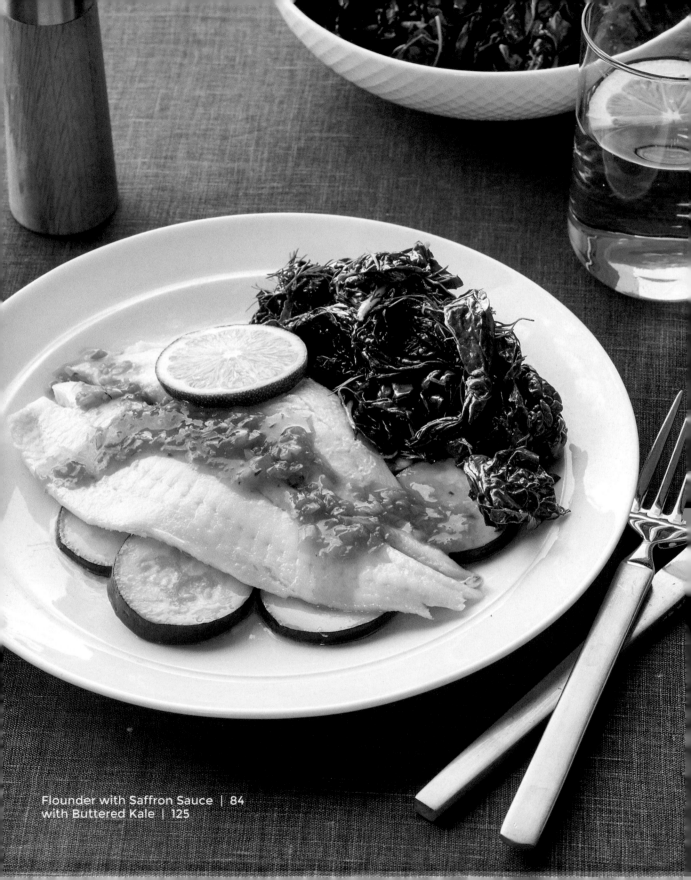

Flounder with Saffron Sauce | 84
with Buttered Kale | 125

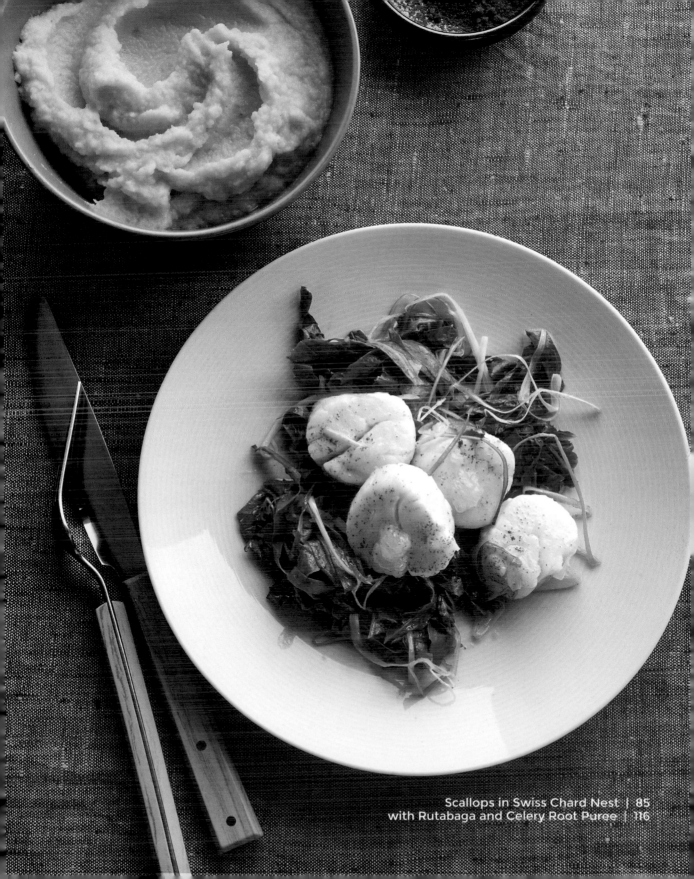

Scallops in Swiss Chard Nest | 85
with Rutabaga and Celery Root Puree | 116

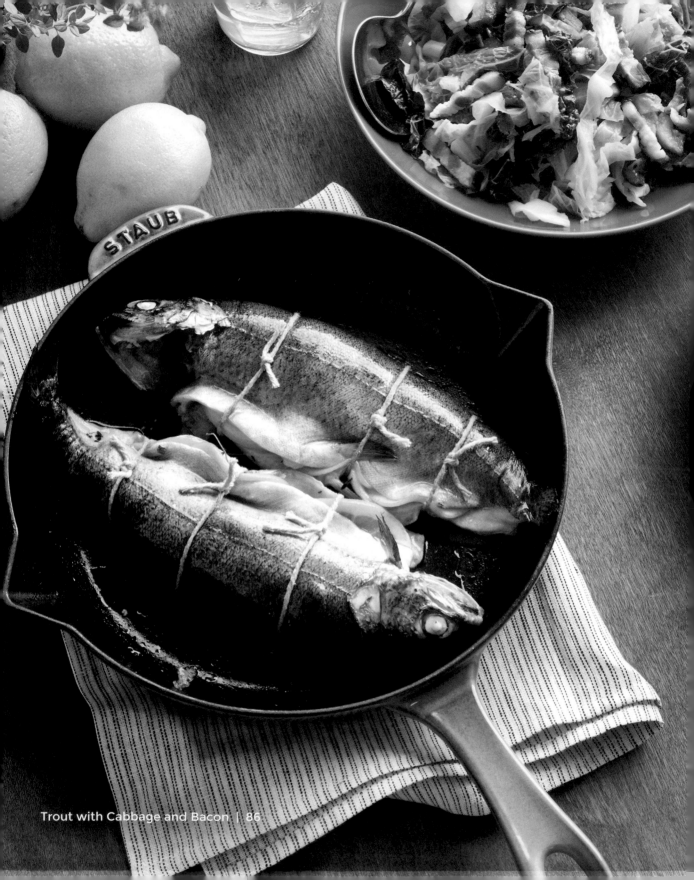

Trout with Cabbage and Bacon | 86

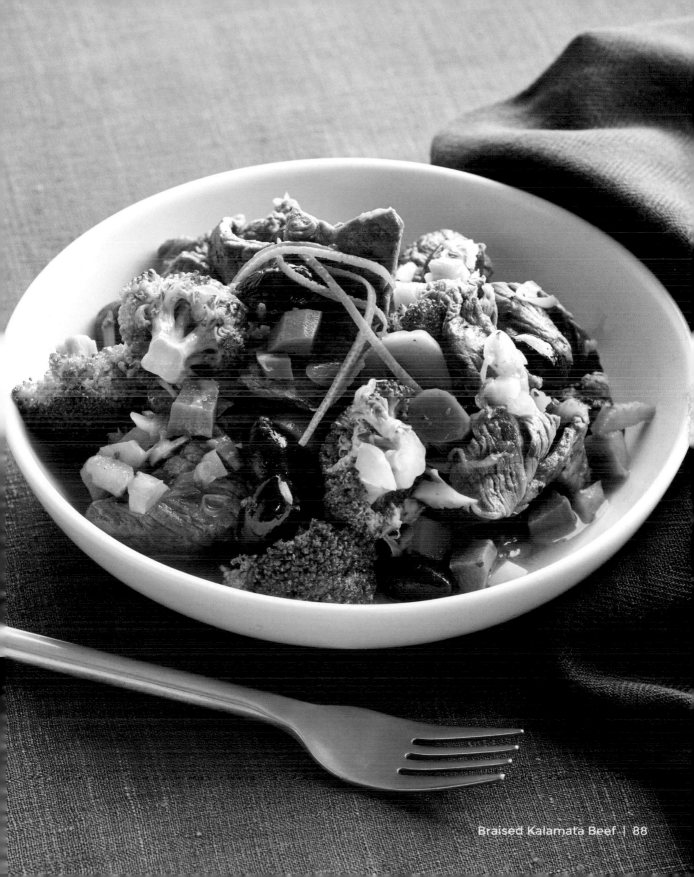

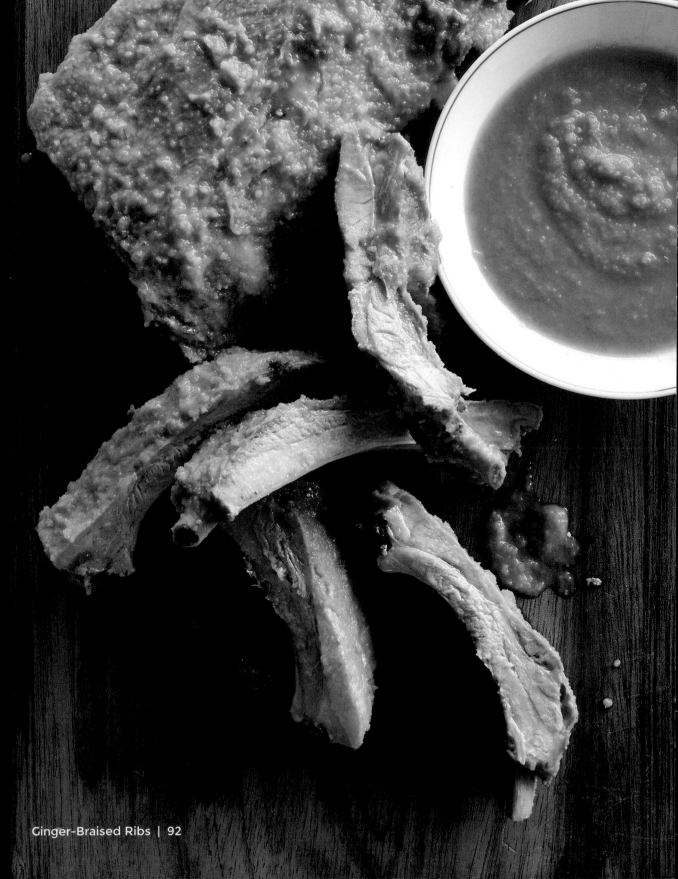

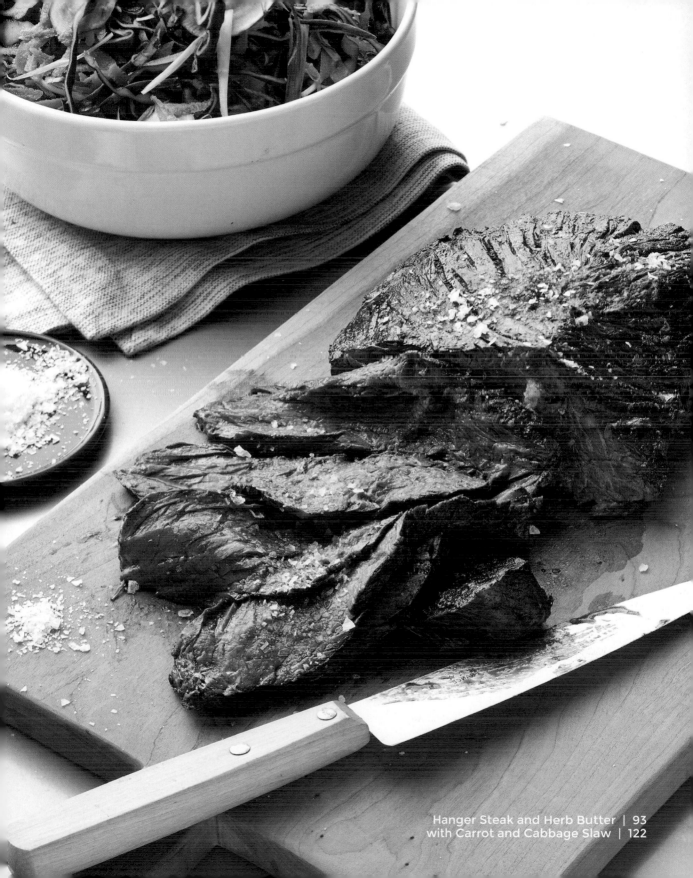

Hanger Steak and Herb Butter | 93
with Carrot and Cabbage Slaw | 122

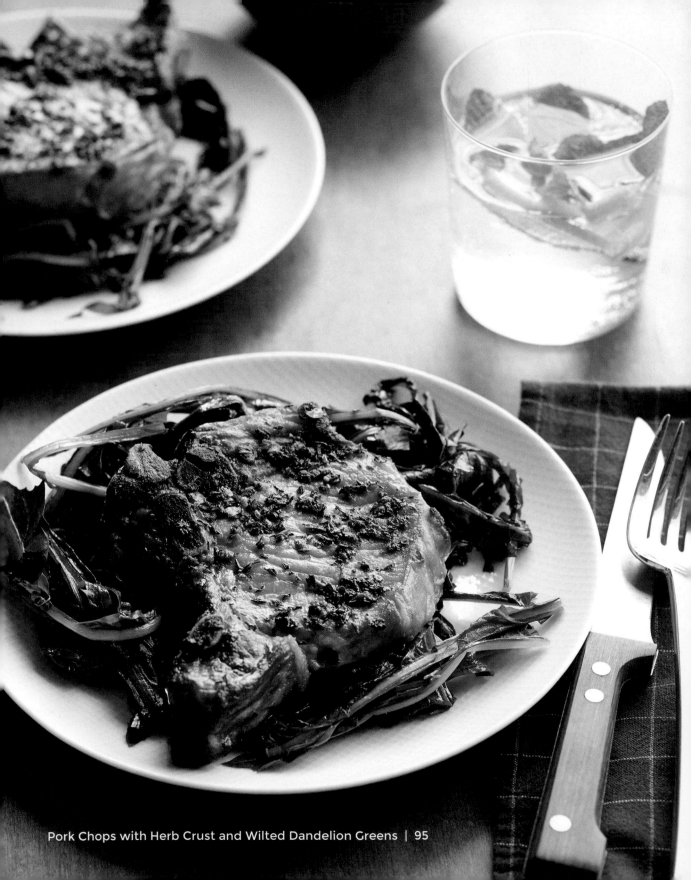

Pork Chops with Herb Crust and Wilted Dandelion Greens | 95

SOLE WITH CELERY PUREE AND GREEN BEANS

SERVES 2

When I spent a little more than a year as a raw vegan, I became an expert in purees. When that lifestyle failed to provide the results I wanted, I became Bulletproof but retained my puree skills, which allowed me to achieve flavors Mother Nature could never match.

4   large stalks celery, cut into 2-inch pieces

1   small leek, trimmed, washed, and quartered

     Sea salt

2   tablespoons grass-fed unsalted butter

2   teaspoons Bulletproof Brain Octane oil (or MCT or coconut oil)

¼   pound green beans

2   sole fillets (½ pound each)

1   tablespoon finely chopped fresh chives

2   teaspoons coarsely chopped fresh tarragon leaves

In a medium saucepan, bring 1 cup water, covered, to a simmer over medium heat. Add the celery and cook, covered, for 3 minutes. Add the leek and a pinch of salt, cover, and cook until the vegetables are tender, about 2 minutes longer. Reserving the pan, transfer the celery and leeks to a blender with ½ cup of the cooking liquid, 1 tablespoon of the butter, and 1 teaspoon of the Brain Octane oil. Puree until well blended. Season with salt to taste and set the puree aside.

Add 1 cup water to the same saucepan, cover, and bring to a simmer. Add the beans and cook until crisp-tender, 3 to 4 minutes. Drain and set aside.

In a large skillet, melt the remaining 1 tablespoon butter with the remaining 1 teaspoon Brain Octane oil over low heat. Add the sole, swirling the pan to coat the fish with the butter/oil. Cover and cook over medium-low heat until just cooked through, 5 to 6 minutes, reducing the heat (if they start to brown) and basting with butter/oil halfway through. Season with sea salt.

To serve, ladle the celery puree into bowls and top with sole and green beans. Drizzle the fish with the remaining butter/oil and sprinkle with chives and tarragon.

FLOUNDER WITH SAFFRON SAUCE

SERVES 2

Saffron used to be one of the most prized, expensive spices in the world. Today it's more accessible and slightly more affordable though still pricey. It's actually the thread of a flower known for having antioxidant properties and carotenoids like lycopene. Some researchers are even studying saffron for anti-cancer benefits.

4	small zucchini (1 pound total), cut into ½-inch-thick rounds
2	flounder fillets (½ pound each)
2	tablespoons Bulletproof Brain Octane oil (or MCT or coconut oil)
	Sea salt
6	tablespoons cold grass-fed unsalted butter
6	lime slices (¼ inch thick)
¼	cup minced leek, white part only
	Scant ¼ teaspoon saffron, crushed
2	kaffir lime leaves
2	tablespoons fresh lime juice
2	tablespoons apple cider vinegar

Preheat the oven to 320°F.

In a 2-quart 8 x 8-inch square baking dish, lay out the zucchini slices and place the flounder on top. Drizzle with the Brain Octane oil, season with sea salt to taste, and top with 2 tablespoons of the butter and the lime slices. Cover and bake until cooked through, 20 to 25 minutes.

Meanwhile, in a small saucepan, combine the leek, saffron, lime leaves, lime juice, and vinegar. Cook over low heat, stirring occasionally, until the leek is soft and there are about 2 tablespoons of liquid left, 5 to 6 minutes. Remove the pan from the heat and whisk in the remaining 4 tablespoons of butter 2 tablespoons at a time. Remove the lime leaves. Season to taste with salt.

Serve the fish and zucchini with the saffron butter sauce.

SCALLOPS IN SWISS CHARD NEST

SERVES 2

Feel free to omit the cayenne if you're nitrate sensitive. You can also try wrapping these with banana leaves (which you'll find in Asian markets or online) for an exotic touch and a burst of flavor. It's easy to double the recipe using a larger baking sheet. I recommend serving this dish with Rutabaga and Celery Root Puree (page 116).

1 bunch Swiss chard (about 12 ounces), large stem ends trimmed, finely sliced

2 scallions, halved crosswise and thinly sliced lengthwise into long threads

1 pound wild sea scallops, tendon removed, and patted dry (no need to rinse)

2 tablespoons Bulletproof Brain Octane oil (or MCT or coconut oil)

3 tablespoons grass-fed unsalted butter or Cilantro-Lime Compound Butter (page 201), cut into 1/2-inch cubes

4 lemon segments (see below), cut into small pieces (1 1/2 tablespoons)

1 teaspoon sea salt (or to taste)

Pinch of cayenne pepper (optional)

4 teaspoons high-quality olive oil

Preheat the oven to 320°F. On a rimmed baking sheet, position two pieces of parchment twice the size of the baking sheet. Dividing evenly, top each piece of parchment with Swiss chard, scallions, and scallops. Top each scallop mixture with the Brain Octane oil and butter, and scatter the lemon pieces on top. Sprinkle with the sea salt and cayenne pepper (if using).

Wrap the scallops and Swiss chard in the parchment, folding seams and tucking in the sides to ensure no steam will escape. Bake until the scallops are medium-rare and the Swiss chard is wilted and tender, 15 to 20 minutes. Open carefully and watch for escaping steam! Drizzle with the olive oil and serve.

HOW TO SEGMENT CITRUS: Cut off the bottom and top of the fruit. Using a chef's knife, cut away the pith and peel leaving the flesh intact. Cut in between the membranes, releasing the fruit and juice into a bowl.

TROUT WITH CABBAGE AND BACON

SERVES 2

Surf and turf usually means lobster and steak, but fish and meat can combine in lots of tasty ways. Here, the bacon and cabbage side dish enhances the delicate flavor of the trout but doesn't overwhelm it.

2	thick-cut slices pastured slab bacon (3 ounces total), cut into $\frac{1}{4}$-inch lardons
6	cups $\frac{1}{2}$-inch-thick strips savoy cabbage
2	sprigs fresh thyme plus 2 teaspoons thyme leaves
$\frac{1}{4}$	cup water
3	tablespoons grass-fed unsalted butter, cut into small pieces
1	tablespoon apple cider vinegar
	Coarse sea salt
2	wild trout (8 to 9 ounces each), cleaned and butterflied by fishmonger
$\frac{1}{2}$	scallion, diced (optional)
6	lemon slices ($\frac{1}{8}$ inch thick), plus juice to taste for serving
2	teaspoons Bulletproof Brain Octane oil (or MCT or coconut oil)

Preheat the oven to 320°F.

In a large, high-sided ovenproof skillet with a lid, cook the bacon over medium-low heat, stirring occasionally, until cooked but not browned, about 5 minutes. Add the cabbage, thyme sprigs, and water. Cover and cook, stirring occasionally, until tender, 8 to 10 minutes. Stir in 1 tablespoon of the butter and the vinegar. Remove the thyme and season with salt to taste. Transfer the cabbage and bacon to a bowl and set aside in a warm place. Wipe out and reserve the skillet.

Place both fish, open, on a cutting board. Top each with 1 tablespoon butter, 1 teaspoon thyme leaves, diced scallion (if using), and salt to taste. Place 3 lemon slices into each fish and close the trout.

Rub the fish with the Brain Octane oil, transfer to the reserved skillet, cover, and bake until just firm and opaque, 18 to 20 minutes. Season to taste with lemon juice and salt.

TROUT NOT-FRIED NOT-RICE

SERVES 2, WITH LEFTOVERS

I always find it hard to believe that I'm eating vegetables with good quality protein in this dish because the cauliflower is so much better than regular rice.

1	cauliflower (1 pound 6 ounces), cut into 2-inch florets
2	large pastured eggs
	Sea salt, to taste
1	tablespoon ghee
1	tablespoon Bulletproof Brain Octane oil (or MCT or coconut oil)
1	scallion, thinly sliced, white and dark green parts kept separate
1	tablespoon minced peeled fresh ginger
¾	teaspoon ground coriander
½	cup grated carrots (about 2 small carrots)
1	celery stalk, cut into ⅛-inch-thick slices (about ½ cup)
3	tablespoons water
2½	ounces smoked trout, flaked
½	teaspoon fresh lime juice

In a food processor, pulse the cauliflower until evenly broken into small grains, working in batches as necessary.

In a small bowl, lightly beat the eggs with salt.

In a large skillet, heat the ghee over medium heat. Add the eggs and swirl to coat the pan. Reduce the heat to medium-low and cook until the eggs are just set, 1 to 2 minutes. Remove the eggs to a plate and slice into thin strips.

Wipe out the pan, return to medium heat, and add the Brrain Octane oil, scallion whites, and ginger. Cook until fragrant, about 30 seconds. Add the coriander, carrots, celery, cauliflower, and water. Cook, stirring constantly, until the vegetables are crisp-tender, about 6 minutes. Stir in the smoked trout, lime juice, egg strips, and scallion greens. Season with salt to taste.

BRAISED KALAMATA BEEF

SERVES 2, WITH LEFTOVERS

Using a tender cut of meat makes it fast to cook this dish, but you can also use a tougher cut and cook it longer for equally enjoyable results.

1 bunch scallions, white and light green parts only, thinly sliced

1 bunch broccoli, stems peeled and finely chopped, florets cut into 1-inch pieces

1 piece (2 inches) fresh ginger, peeled and thinly sliced

1 orange

1 pound boneless grass-fed sirloin, thinly sliced

½ cup Kalamata olives, pitted

1 carrot, coarsely chopped

½ cup water

1 teaspoon apple cider vinegar

1 tablespoon dried oregano

1 bay leaf

1 teaspoon coarse sea salt

1 tablespoon chopped parsley leaves

½ cup ghee or grass-fed unsalted butter

1 tablespoon Bulletproof Brain Octane oil (or MCT or coconut oil)

1 tablespoon sesame oil

In a Dutch oven or large pot, combine the white parts of the scallions, broccoli stems, and ginger and cook over low heat until fragrant, about 5 minutes.

Meanwhile, grate 1 teaspoon of zest from the orange (set the zest aside). Then peel and segment the orange (see How to Segment Citrus, page 85).

Add the broccoli florets, orange segments, beef, olives, carrot, water, vinegar, oregano, bay leaf, and salt to the pot. Cover and cook until the beef is tender and the vegetables are crisp tender, at least 10 minutes. Stir in the green parts of the scallions, the orange zest, parsley, ghee, Brain Octane oil, and sesame oil.

BRAISED NO-CHILE LAMB CHILI

SERVES 2, WITH LEFTOVERS

You'd be amazed how many people are sensitive to nightshades. This recipe eliminates those ingredients that can take quality out of your day by using a high-quality seasoning blend instead of peppers.

1 leek, well washed and thinly sliced

2 carrots, finely chopped

4 celery stalks, thinly sliced

2 cups water

½ cup thinly sliced asparagus

1 cup chopped cauliflower

1 cup chopped zucchini and/or summer squash

1 pound ground pastured lamb

1 teaspoon apple cider vinegar

1 teaspoon coriander seeds

1 teaspoon cumin seeds

1 teaspoon allspice berries

1 teaspoon ground annatto (achiote)

1 tablespoon dried oregano

1 bay leaf

1 teaspoon coarse sea salt

¼ cup coconut oil

1 tablespoon Bulletproof Brain Octane oil (or MCT or coconut oil)

High-quality olive oil, for drizzling

In a medium pot, combine the leek, carrots, and celery and cook over medium-low heat until fragrant and the leek is soft, about 3 minutes. Add the water, asparagus, cauliflower, zucchini, lamb, vinegar, spices, oregano, bay leaf, and sea salt. Cover and cook until the lamb is cooked through and the vegetables are just tender, about 10 minutes. Stir in the coconut oil, Brain Octane oil, and a drizzle of olive oil.

BEEF CHILI

SERVES 2, WITH LEFTOVERS

I grew up in New Mexico where chili was made differently than in other regions. This version is a sort of Texas-style chili, but I use butternut squash, which tastes amazing. Try this dish with an avocado slice and a squeeze of lime. Any leftovers will make a great lunch served over a baked sweet potato. Just be sure you use high-quality chili powder and cayenne if you opt to use them. And if you're one of those people to whom cilantro tastes like soap, it's no problem to skip it.

¾ teaspoon Bulletproof Brain Octane oil (or MCT or coconut oil)

2 slices thick-cut pastured slab bacon, cut into ¼-inch lardons

1 small carrot, grated

½ cup finely chopped leek

1 pound ground grass-fed beef

1 teaspoon ground cumin

1 teaspoon ground coriander

1¼ teaspoons chili powder or cayenne (optional)

1 teaspoon ground cinnamon

1 bay leaf

Coarse sea salt

1¼ cups water

2 cups peeled and diced butternut squash

¼ cup coarsely chopped fresh cilantro leaves

In a medium saucepan, heat the Brain Octane oil and bacon over medium heat. Cook, stirring often, taking care not to char the bacon, until it is firm but tender, about 2 minutes. Add the carrot and leek and cook, stirring, for 1 minute. Add the beef, cumin, coriander, chili powder (if using), cinnamon, bay leaf, and a good pinch of sea salt. Cook, breaking apart the meat, until it is firm and golden, about 3 minutes.

Add the water and bring to a simmer. Cover, reduce the heat to low, and cook for 20 minutes. Add the squash and cook until the squash is tender, 8 to 10 minutes. Discard the bay leaf and season the chili with salt to taste. Garnish with the cilantro.

PORK FLANK STEAK WITH COCONUT RELISH

For years, I avoided pork because I thought it was somehow bad or unhealthy. It turns out that the quality of the pork is the most important thing. With quality meat, this is an amazing dish. Pastured pork flank is a flavorful cut available from a butcher or farmers' market that supplies pork belly. Lightly grilling it is a great option, as the steaks are thin and you won't risk charring the meat so it's both tasty and toxin-free.

1	scallion, minced
¼	cup finely chopped fresh basil
¼	cup chopped fresh cilantro
1	tablespoon chopped fresh oregano leaves
½	teaspoon ground cumin
1	teaspoon grated peeled fresh ginger
2	tablespoons unsweetened coconut flakes, finely chopped
2	tablespoons high-quality olive oil
3	tablespoons Bulletproof Brain Octane oil (or MCT or coconut oil)
2	tablespoons apple cider vinegar
	Coarse sea salt
4	pastured pork flank steaks (about 3½ ounces each)

Heat a grill pan over (or fire up your grill to) medium-high heat.

In a small bowl, combine the scallion, basil, cilantro, oregano, cumin, ginger, coconut flakes, olive oil, 2 tablespoons Brain Octane oil, the vinegar, and 1 teaspoon salt. Stir the coconut relish well to combine.

Rub all the steaks with the remaining 1 tablespoon Brain Octane oil and sprinkle with sea salt. Place the steaks on the grill, reduce the heat to medium-low, and grill briefly, taking care not to char the meat, for 4 to 5 minutes per side for rare and 5 to 6 minutes per side for medium-rare. Remove the steaks to a cutting board, allow to rest for 5 minutes, then thinly slice against the grain.

Serve the steak topped with the coconut relish.

GINGER-BRAISED RIBS

SERVES 2, WITH LEFTOVERS

If you've been on a low-fat diet before, you've probably gazed longingly at ribs and thought you'd never enjoy their tender juiciness again. This recipe makes it possible. Beta-carotene and fiber-rich carrots serve as a base for the barbecue sauce so it's nutrient dense as well as delicious.

1¾	pounds pastured baby back pork ribs
1½	cups water
¼	cup chopped leek, white part only
5	small carrots, trimmed and left whole
1	piece (3 inches) fresh ginger, peeled and cut into thirds
1	sprig fresh oregano
3	tablespoons apple cider vinegar
3	tablespoons xylitol
	Sea salt

Preheat the oven to 300°F.

Place the ribs, water, leek, carrots, ginger, and oregano in the bottom of a 9 x 13-inch baking pan. Cover with foil and bake until the carrots and ribs are just tender, 1 hour 30 minutes to 1 hour 45 minutes. Leave the oven on.

Discard the oregano. Transfer the ribs to a dish and set aside. Transfer the carrots, ginger, leek, and braising liquid to a food processor or blender and puree until smooth. Blend in the vinegar and xylitol. Season with salt to taste. Return the ribs and the sauce to the baking pan. Pour the carrot sauce over the ribs and turn once to coat. Cover with foil and bake, basting with sauce once halfway through cooking, until the ribs are tender when pierced with a knife and the sauce is thickened, 30 to 40 minutes. Slice the ribs and serve with the pan sauce.

HANGER STEAK AND HERB BUTTER

SERVES 2

I've always liked the quick convenient nature of this dish, which is great for lunch or dinner. You could also use a strip steak for convenience or put the herb butter on a ribeye.

- 1 hanger steak ($\frac{1}{2}$ pound)
- 1 tablespoon Bulletproof Brain Octane oil (or MCT or coconut oil)
- 1 lemon
- 4 tablespoons (2 ounces) grass-fed unsalted butter, at room temperature
- 1 tablespoon minced chives
- 2 tablespoons mixed chopped fresh herbs (oregano, thyme, or rosemary)

  Sea salt
- 3 cups (about 3 ounces) spinach

Rub the steak with the Brain Octane oil and set aside.

Grate 2 teaspoons of zest from the lemon. Halve the lemon and cut into wedges. Squeeze out 1 teaspoon of juice and set the remaining lemon wedges aside.

In a small bowl, combine the lemon zest, butter, chives, herbs, and 1 teaspoon sea salt, stirring well to combine and create a compound butter. Stir in the lemon juice.

Heat a grill pan over (or fire up your grill to) medium-high heat. Season the steak with sea salt, place on the grill, and reduce the heat to medium-low. Cook, taking care not to char the meat, for 5 to 6 minutes per side for rare, 6 to 7 minutes per side for medium-rare. Transfer the steak to a plate, top with 2$\frac{1}{2}$ tablespoons compound butter (reserve remaining compound butter for another use), and allow to rest for 5 minutes. Slice the steak thinly across the grain, and serve with the spinach, topping with meat juices and a squeeze of lemon.

PORK BELLY CILANTRO STEW

SERVES 2

Honestly, 10 years ago, I knew nothing about pork belly. Once I experienced it, I was blown away at the difference between this pork product and bacon. Serve it with Carrot and Sweet Potato Mash (page 127) or Cauliflower "Couscous" (page 117).

2	teaspoons Bulletproof Brain Octane oil (or MCT or coconut oil)
1	pound pastured pork belly, cut into 1-inch pieces
1	small leek, well washed, white and light green parts only, cut into $\frac{1}{2}$-inch chunks (about 1 cup)
1	tablespoon minced fresh ginger
2	teaspoons fresh oregano leaves
$\frac{1}{2}$	cup apple cider vinegar
$\frac{1}{2}$	cup canned coconut milk, well shaken
2	bay leaves, fresh is best
$\frac{3}{4}$	teaspoon coarse sea salt
1	bunch cilantro ($2\frac{1}{2}$ ounces), leaves picked ($1\frac{1}{4}$ packed cups)

In a medium saucepan, melt the Brain Octane oil over medium-low heat. Add the pork belly and cook gently, turning every 2 minutes, until just browned, about 10 minutes.

Add the leek, ginger, oregano, vinegar, coconut milk, bay leaves, and salt. Stir to combine. Bring the mixture to a low simmer, then cover and cook until the pork belly is tender when pierced with a knife, 45 to 50 minutes. Let cool for 10 minutes, then spoon the fat off the surface and reserve. Measure out and set aside 2 tablespoons of fat for the sauce.

Use a slotted spoon to transfer the pork belly to a dish. Remove the bay leaves and transfer the sauce to a blender. Add the cilantro and the 2 tablespoons reserved fat, and puree to a fine, bright-green sauce.

Serve the pork belly topped with the cilantro sauce.

PORK CHOPS WITH HERB CRUST AND WILTED DANDELION GREENS

SERVES 2

If you've never eaten dandelion because it's a weed, you're not alone. But if you can find them, try them. Yes, they're bitter, but they cut the rich fat flavor profile of the pork chop. Also, they're rich in beta-carotene, B vitamins, and potassium.

- 1 tablespoon *each* minced fresh parsley, oregano, sage, and thyme
  Sea salt
- 2 bone-in pastured pork chops ($\frac{1}{2}$ inch thick, 6 to 8 ounces each)
- 1 teaspoon Bulletproof Brain Octane oil (or MCT or coconut oil)
- $1\frac{1}{2}$ tablespoons grass-fed unsalted butter
- 1 bunch dandelion greens, trimmed, washed, and roughly chopped

In a small bowl, combine the herbs and 1 teaspoon salt. Coat both sides of the pork chops with the herb mixture.

Heat a heavy pan such as a cast-iron skillet over medium heat. Add the oil and the chops. Reduce the heat if the meat is in danger of charring. Cook gently until the chops are golden, but not browned, 4 to 5 minutes per side. Remove the pan from the heat and add the butter, turning the chops to coat. Remove the chops to a plate and add the dandelion greens to the reserved pan. Cook, tossing once, for 2 minutes. Season with salt to taste.

BRAISED LAMB WITH SAFFRON AND GINGER

SERVES 2, WITH LEFTOVERS

When I was growing up, it was only on rare occasions that we ate lamb.
Now I buy a whole lamb from the people that raise it. I know that it's tender
and flavorful and not gamey at all. Braising is a great Bulletproof technique
that keeps all the nutrients intact—just remember to cook it slow and low so
you don't risk overcooking the meat.

1 tablespoon plus 1 teaspoon ghee

2 pounds boneless pastured lamb shoulder, cut into 1-inch pieces

3 whole cardamom pods

1 piece (3 inches) fresh ginger, peeled and minced

Pinch of saffron, crushed

1 teaspoon ground turmeric

1 cinnamon stick

2½ cups beef stock or Upgraded Bone Broth (page 147)

Sea salt

4 carrots, cut into ½-inch pieces

1 tablespoon finely grated orange zest, for serving

Fresh cilantro leaves, for serving

1 teaspoon raw honey (optional), for serving

Preheat the oven to 320°F.

In a large ovenproof pot or Dutch oven, melt the ghee over medium heat. Add the
lamb and cook, turning once or twice, until the outside of the meat is just cooked, about
8 minutes. Add the cardamom, ginger, saffron, turmeric, cinnamon stick, stock or broth,
and salt to taste. Cover and transfer to the oven.

Bake until the lamb is almost tender, about 1 hour 20 minutes. Add the carrots and
continue to cook until tender, 15 to 20 minutes longer. Garnish with the orange zest,
cilantro, and honey (if using).

LAMB WITH CUMIN AND SUMAC

SERVES 2

Cumin may not be the most familiar spice to some, but here it stands out and shines. When you try this recipe, you'll be amazed at how the spice comes through and enhances the lamb. Serve this with the Cauliflower "Couscous" (page 117).

1 pound boneless pastured lamb leg or shoulder, cut into 1½-inch pieces

3 teaspoons Bulletproof Brain Octane oil (or MCT or coconut oil)

½ teaspoon *each* ground cumin, sumac, and allspice

1 tablespoon *each* minced fresh cilantro, oregano, and mint

1 teaspoon coarse sea salt

In a medium bowl, combine the lamb, 2 teaspoons of the oil, the cumin, sumac, allspice, cilantro, oregano, mint, and sea salt, stirring to coat. Cover and refrigerate for at least 1 hour and up to 4 hours.

In a large skillet, heat the remaining 1 teaspoon oil over medium heat. Add the lamb and cook, turning to brown on all sides, but taking care not to char it, until medium-rare, 7 to 8 minutes.

NOTE: You can also thread the lamb onto skewers and grill the meat, without charring, turning occasionally over medium heat, for 8 to 9 minutes, until medium-rare.

DUCK CONFIT

SERVES 2

The first time I went to France, in the 1990s, I didn't know what duck confit was. Then I tried it and became obsessed. Of course it's full of duck fat so it tastes amazing, with a better health profile than chicken meat. Your best choice is to use pastured ducks that are free of antibiotics. And be sure to save the leftover strained duck fat; it's great for using on Carrot and Sweet Potato Mash (page 127).

2	duck legs or 2 duck breasts (from a 5-pound pastured duck)
1½	teaspoons coarse sea salt
1	tablespoon fresh thyme leaves
2	teaspoons fresh oregano leaves
4	cups duck fat, available at farmers' markets or specialty butcher shops

Preheat the oven to 300°F.

Score the duck breasts, if using. Combine the salt, thyme, and oregano in a small bowl. Rub the duck with the herb-salt. Cover and refrigerate for 8 hours.

In a small pot, melt the duck fat over low heat until liquid. Scrape as much of herb-salt off the duck as possible. Submerge the duck in the fat, cover, and cook until tender, about 1 hour for the duck breasts and 1 hour 30 minutes for the legs.

Store the duck completely submerged in the strained fat in the refrigerator for up to 1 month.

To use, remove the duck from the fat and reheat gently in a 320°F oven until warmed through and the skin is lightly golden, 10 to 12 minutes. (The strained fat can be saved and frozen for up to 3 months.)

WINTER SQUASH AND SWEET POTATO "RISOTTO"

SERVES 2

If you're used to a high-carb diet, you surely love the creamy, fatty taste and texture of risotto. When you make this version, subbing in sweet potato, you enjoy the same sensation with a slightly different flavor. Add Pork Chops with Herb Crust (page 95) or steak and you'll be in heaven. To enhance the resemblance to risotto, dice the squash and potato very fine and reduce the cooking time.

1	tablespoon ghee or grass-fed unsalted butter
1	tablespoon Bulletproof Brain Octane oil (or MCT or coconut oil)
1	small leek, white part only, diced (optional)
2½	cups peeled, diced (½-inch) butternut squash
2½	cups peeled, diced (½-inch) sweet potato
1	teaspoon fresh thyme leaves
1	teaspoon fresh oregano leaves
1	cup Upgraded Bone Broth (page 147)
	Sea salt

In a medium saucepan, melt the ghee in the Brain Octane oil over medium-low heat. Add the leek (if using) and cook, stirring, for 1 minute, taking care not to brown it. Add the squash, sweet potato, and herbs, stirring once to combine. Add the broth and season with salt to taste. Simmer gently, stirring occasionally, until the sweet potato is soft and the squash is just tender, 18 to 20 minutes. Adjust the salt to taste. Serve warm.

BULLETPROOF CEVICHE

SERVES 1

This dish is easily adaptable to other varieties of wild-caught mercury-free Bulletproof fish; try it with fluke. Make it after lunch and it will be well cured by dinnertime. Enjoy it with some watercress or arugula and a drizzle of lime juice and Brain Octane oil.

8	ounces wild boneless, skinless salmon fillet, cut into $1/2$-inch dice
2	tablespoons fresh lime juice
1	teaspoon high-quality olive oil
1	teaspoon Bulletproof Brain Octane oil (or MCT or coconut oil)
$1/2$	avocado, pitted, peeled, and cut into $1/2$-inch dice
1	scallion, thinly sliced
1	tablespoon fresh cilantro leaves, torn, plus more for garnish
	Sea salt

In a medium bowl, toss the fish with lime juice, olive oil, and Brain Octane oil. Fold in the avocado, scallion, and cilantro, mixing well to combine. Season with sea salt to taste. Refrigerate, stirring every 15 minutes to distribute the lime juice, for at least 2 hours. More marinating time is fine, as long as it's in the refrigerator. Garnish with cilantro to serve.

WARM LAMB AND CHICKPEA SALAD

SERVES 2, WITH LEFTOVERS

The seasoned lamb mixture also makes great meatballs: Crack 1 large egg into the mix, form into meatballs, and bake at 320°F until just cooked through.

- 1 teaspoon ground cumin
- 1/2 teaspoon ground cinnamon
- 1/2 teaspoon ground allspice
- 1 teaspoon finely chopped fresh oregano
- 1 scallion, finely chopped
- 1 pound ground lamb
- 1/3 cup mixed chopped fresh herbs: parsley, mint, and/or cilantro
  Sea salt
  Grated zest of 1 lemon
- 1 tablespoon fresh lemon juice
- 1 tablespoon high-quality olive oil
- 2 tablespoons Bulletproof Brain Octane oil (or MCT or coconut oil)
- 2 cups cooked chickpeas
  Radicchio, halved, cored, and leaves separated, for serving

In a large bowl, combine the cumin, cinnamon, allspice, oregano, scallion, lamb, mixed herbs, and 1 teaspoon salt. Use clean hands to mix well to combine. Marinate the lamb-mixture for 1 hour in the refrigerator.

In a large bowl, combine the lemon zest, lemon juice, olive oil, and 1 tablespoon of the Brain Octane oil. Add the chickpeas and toss. Season with salt to taste.

In a large skillet, heat the remaining 1 tablespoon Brain Octane oil over medium heat until shimmering. Add the lamb and cook without browning, breaking the lamb into pieces until cooked through, about 5 minutes.

Add the lamb to the bowl with the chickpeas and toss to combine. Serve immediately with radicchio leaves.

BULLETPROOF ROAST SIRLOIN WITH BRUSSELS SPROUTS

SERVES 2 TO 4

For this recipe you'll need a slow cooker, which is on the "suspect list" because people tend to use it to overcook things. Used correctly, on "low" as here, it's a great tool that I recommend for making lots of Bulletproof dishes with minimal effort.

Roast

- 1 pound grass-fed bottom sirloin or skirt steak
- 2 tablespoons coarse sea salt
- 1 tablespoon ground turmeric
- 1 teaspoon dried oregano
- 2 tablespoons Bulletproof Brain Octane oil (or MCT or coconut oil)
- 3 tablespoons grass-fed unsalted butter
- 1½ tablespoons apple cider vinegar

Brussels Sprouts

- 1 pound Brussels sprouts, halved
- 2 tablespoons grass-fed unsalted butter
- 2 teaspoons fine sea salt
- 2 teaspoons ground turmeric

For the roast: Rub the meat with the salt, turmeric, and oregano. Place the seasoned meat in the slow cooker and pour on the Brain Octane oil. Add the butter, cover, and slow-cook on low for 6 to 8 hours, or until the meat is shreddable. After the meat is cooked, add the vinegar.

For the Brussels sprouts: Preheat the oven to 300°F.

Spread the Brussels sprouts on a baking sheet and dot with the butter. Sprinkle on the salt and turmeric. Bake until fork-tender, 30 to 45 minutes. Serve and enjoy.

ALL-IN-ONE TURKEY BURGERS

MAKES 4 BURGERS

Keep your total poultry consumption to once or twice a week when you are in maintenance mode. This burger packs protein, vegetables, and a host of saturated fats. Pair with the Carrot and Cabbage Slaw (page 122) or the Braised Romaine and Endive (page 134).

1½	pounds ground dark meat pastured turkey
2	slices thick-cut pastured bacon, cut into ¼-inch dice
½	cup packed fresh cilantro leaves, chopped
1	scallion, minced
½	cup shredded zucchini
1	large pastured egg yolk
2¼	teaspoons chopped fresh thyme leaves
1	teaspoon ground cumin
½	teaspoon ground allspice
½	teaspoon ground ginger
1	tablespoon high-quality olive oil
2	tablespoons Bulletproof Brain Octane oil (or MCT or coconut oil)
1	teaspoon coarse sea salt

Preheat the oven to 325°F. Line a baking sheet with parchment paper.

In a large bowl, combine the turkey, bacon, cilantro, scallion, zucchini, egg yolk, thyme, cumin, allspice, ginger, olive oil, 1 tablespoon of the Brain Octane oil, and the sea salt. Mix well until combined. Form into 4 patties and place on the baking sheet. Drizzle with the remaining 1 tablespoon Brain Octane oil.

Bake, uncovered, until the burgers are cooked through and register an internal temperature of 165°F, 35 to 40 minutes.

BULLETPROOF CHICKEN

SERVES 2, PLUS LEFTOVERS

Poultry fat is high in omega-6s, so limit your poultry consumption to once or twice a week at most and make sure your chicken is local and pastured to avoid a GMO-fed bird. When preparing the herbs and vegetables for this chicken, save the trimmings, stems, and peels to add to a stock later (or for a future bone or beef broth). I save mine in the freezer so I have them on hand the next time I need to make stock in a hurry.

3	tablespoons ghee, at room temperature
¼	cup chopped fresh parsley
10	fresh sage leaves, minced (about 1½ tablespoons)
1	tablespoon minced fresh chives
1	tablespoon chopped fresh oregano leaves
1	tablespoon fresh thyme leaves
2	teaspoons grated lemon zest
	Coarse sea salt
4	medium carrots, cut into 1½- to 2-inch lengths
1½	teaspoons Bulletproof Brain Octane oil (or MCT or coconut oil)
1	whole organic pastured chicken (3½ pounds), patted dry
	One 2-inch length of leek, trimmed, rinsed, and halved

Preheat the oven to 325°F.

In a small bowl, stir together the ghee, herbs, lemon zest, and 1 teaspoon salt. Measure out and set aside 1 tablespoon of the herbed ghee for basting.

In a Dutch oven or large pot, combine the carrots and ½ teaspoon of the Brain Octane oil and toss. Dot with half the herbed ghee remaining in the small bowls.

Pat the chicken dry and loosen the skin around the breast and thighs. Spread the last of the herbed ghee from the small bowl under the skin of the breast and thighs. Tuck the wing tips under the chicken thighs and place the leek inside the cavity of the chicken. Tie the legs together with kitchen twine. Rub the outside of the chicken with the remaining 1 teaspoon Brain Octane oil and sprinkle with sea salt.

Place the chicken breast-side up on top of the carrots in the Dutch oven and roast, uncovered, for 1 hour. Baste the chicken with the reserved tablespoon of herbed ghee and return to the oven. Roast until the internal temperature of the chicken registers 165°F and the juices run clear when the thickest part of the thigh is pierced with a knife, 35 to 40 minutes. Allow the chicken to rest for 15 minutes before carving.

COCONUT-BRAISED MACKEREL AND QUICK-PICKLED CARROTS

SERVES 2

Atlantic mackerel is high in omega-3s and lower in mercury than king mackerel or Spanish mackerel. This preparation requires most of the cooking to be done on the skin side, preserving the nutrients in the fish without charring; it simmers gently in curried coconut milk to finish cooking. You can make the pickled carrots ahead of time. And instead of pan-braising the mackerel, as here, you could simply broil or grill it (just be sure to lightly grill and not char the skin or fish).

- $\frac{1}{3}$ cup apple cider vinegar
- 2 tablespoons erythritol
- 2 tablespoons julienned peeled fresh ginger
- 3 allspice berries

  Coarse sea salt
- 2 carrots, cut into 3-inch-long matchsticks
- 2 teaspoons Bulletproof Brain Octane oil (or MCT or coconut oil)
- 2 mackerel fillets (about 6 ounces each), skin scored
- $\frac{1}{2}$ cup canned coconut milk, well shaken
- 1 teaspoon Bulletproof Curry Powder (page 202)
- 3 cups spinach, thinly sliced
- 1 teaspoon fresh lime juice

  Fresh cilantro leaves, for serving

In a small saucepot, combine the vinegar, erythritol, ginger, allspice berries, and 1½ teaspoons salt and bring to a simmer over medium heat. Cook until the salt and erythritol dissolve, about 2 minutes. Add the carrots and reduce the heat to low. Cover and cook until the carrots are crisp-tender, 8 to 10 minutes. Set the carrots aside and discard the allspice.

In a large skillet, heat the Brain Octane oil over medium heat. Add the mackerel, skin-side down, and immediately reduce the heat to medium-low. Cook gently until the skin releases from the pan and the bottom of the fillet is opaque, about 10 minutes.

Season the fish with salt and flip over. Add the coconut milk and curry, swirling to combine. Add the spinach, then cover and cook until the spinach is just wilted, the mackerel is cooked through, and the sauce is reduced slightly, about 3 minutes. Season with the lime juice and sea salt to taste.

Serve with the pickled carrots and cilantro leaves.

CHESTNUT DUMPLINGS WITH ARUGULA AND SQUASH

SERVES 2

A light hand is key when handling the dumpling dough and adding the rice flour. A great meal option for when you are carb re-feeding.

- 3 tablespoons grass-fed unsalted butter, melted
- 5 ounces organic chestnuts, steamed and peeled
- 6 tablespoons water
- 2 tablespoons Bulletproof Brain Octane oil (or MCT or coconut oil)
- Sea salt
- 2 large pastured eggs

- Pinch of cayenne powder (optional)
- 12 tablespoons sweet rice flour, plus more for dusting
- 8 ounces butternut squash, peeled, seeded, and cut into ¼-inch wedges
- 1 to 2 teaspoons lemon juice
- 1 cup arugula
- Lemon wedges, for serving

Bring a large pot of water to a boil.

In a medium saucepan, melt the butter and set aside.

In a food processor, combine the chestnuts, water, Brain Octane oil, and ½ teaspoon salt. Puree until smooth. Measure out ½ cup and transfer to a large bowl (reserve the remaining puree for another use).

Add the eggs and cayenne (if using) to the ½ cup chestnut mixture and whisk together. With a wooden spoon, stir in the rice flour 1 tablespoon at a time until a tacky dough forms. Dust lightly with another tablespoon of flour and roll into two 12-inch-long ropes. Cut the ropes crosswise into 1-inch dumplings.

Salt the boiling water and add the squash. Reduce the heat to a hearty simmer and cook until the squash is just tender, 5 to 7 minutes. With a slotted spoon, transfer the squash to a plate and reserve the pot and cooking water.

Return the water to a boil and add the dumplings. Cook until the dumplings float to the surface, 2 to 3 minutes. Transfer the dumplings to the pan with the melted butter and heat gently over medium heat until simmering; add the lemon juice, turning to coat.

Arrange the squash either alongside or on a bed of arugula and top with the butter-coated dumplings. Serve with lemon wedges for squeezing.

STUFFED SWEET POTATO

SERVES 1

This sweet potato has been upgraded from accompaniment to main-course attraction with the addition of your choice of Bulletproof meat. You can use some of the thinly sliced pork belly from page 94, chopped bacon, or shredded Duck Confit (page 98). If using the duck, you can substitute 2 teaspoons of melted duck fat for the butter. Serve with a side of greens and your choice of Bulletproof dressing.

1   sweet potato, scrubbed and pierced several times with a knife

2   teaspoons grass-fed unsalted butter or Cilantro-Lime Compound Butter (page 201)

¼   cup chopped or shredded Bulletproof meat of your choice

2   teaspoons chopped fresh herbs: oregano, chives, parsley, or cilantro

Sea salt

Preheat the oven to 325°F.

Wrap the sweet potato in foil and place on a rimmed baking sheet. Bake until just tender when pierced with a fork, 1 hour to 1 hour 15 minutes.

Unwrap the sweet potato. Cut a lengthwise slit on top of the sweet potato, pinch the sides, keeping the bottom intact, and top with butter and your choice of Bulletproof meat. Sprinkle with the herbs and sea salt to taste.

CHAPTER 6

SIDES AND SALADS

When I created these side dishes and salads, I designed them to be just as satisfying when enjoyed as standalone meals. They are very versatile; they're great as a late lunch, and they can easily accompany a main dish for a heartier meal. If you're protein fasting or coming out of ketosis, there are plenty of options here to help you stay on track. These dishes were also designed to be good vehicles for your leftover mains; because most every recipe is sized for two, you can either make an easy meal for yourself and someone else, or eat solo and save what's left for lunch the next day. Being Bulletproof makes it easy to keep things efficient and purposeful.

One of my favorite pairings is Curried Cauliflower Steak (right) and Coconut Creamed Spinach (page 114) for a great low-protein entrée. The Braised Radishes and Greens (page 115) alongside the Rutabaga and Celery Root Puree (page 116) make a great combo, too; the creaminess of the puree offsets the bitter radishes. And don't be surprised to see "couscous" in this chapter—it's a grain-free hack that relies on the versatile texture of cauliflower. The Cauliflower "Couscous" (page 117) paired with Broccoli with Tapenade and Bacon (page 130) makes for a nutrient-packed pairing: Both are cruciferous vegetables (leafy veggies with cross-shaped flowers, also known as brassicas, botanically) and they make fine plate-fellows. I like to pile the broccoli atop the couscous. Another vegetable that works beautifully with either the cauliflower steak or the couscous is Spice-Roasted Fennel (page 119). You can also think about pairing the marinated artichokes from the Steamed Artichokes with Salmon and Vinaigrette recipe (page 123) with another side or salad because the portion size is small. I wanted to be mindful of the cost associated with buying fresh artichokes, so this is one of the lighter sides.

Every meal and every side is designed to stretch, so your time is well spent and your energy is rewarded. Get creative and combine these with the main-dish lunches and dinners, other sides and salads, and even warm smoothies for satisfying Bulletproof meals that are never boring.

CURRIED CAULIFLOWER STEAK

SERVES 2

Cauliflower is my all-time favorite vegetable because you can do so much with it, and it maintains a great structure to hold up to all those good fats. I like this with the Coconut Creamed Spinach (page 114) as a great option when you're Bulletproof protein fasting. It's a great combination of two flavorful sides packed with healthy fats.

- 1   head cauliflower, sliced vertically through the core into 1-inch-thick "steaks"
- 2   tablespoons Bulletproof Brain Octane oil (or MCT or coconut oil)
- 2   teaspoons Bulletproof Curry Powder (page 202)
     Sea salt
- 1   tablespoon Cilantro-Lime Compound Butter (page 201)

Preheat the oven to 320°F.

Line a baking sheet with two 24-inch-long pieces of parchment paper. Cross the papers to form a plus sign and set aside. Keeping the cauliflower steaks intact, gently rub them with the Brain Octane oil, curry powder, and sea salt to taste. Wrap the parchment around cauliflower like a package, folding seams, tucking the ends under, and putting seam-side down so no steam escapes. Bake until the cauliflower is just tender, about 35 minutes. Top with the compound butter and serve.

COCONUT CREAMED SPINACH

SERVES 1 OR 2

You'll be surprised how well the flavors of coconut and spinach go together. This recipe can be paired with the Perfect Parchment-Baked Salmon (page 77) or, when you are Bulletproof protein fasting, try it with Curried Cauliflower Steaks (page 113). For an even creamier creamed spinach, pulse it in the food processor until pureed.

1	teaspoon Bulletproof Brain Octane oil (or MCT or coconut oil)
1	small leek, well washed and diced
¾	cup canned coconut milk, well shaken
6	ounces spinach leaves
	Sea salt

In a medium saucepan, gently heat the Brain Octane oil over medium heat. Add the leek and cook, stirring, until translucent and tender, about 3 minutes. Add the coconut milk and bring to a simmer, about 3 minutes. Add the spinach and cook until just wilted, 2 to 3 minutes. Season with sea salt to taste.

BRAISED RADISHES AND GREENS

SERVES 2

This recipe is full of great flavor. Radishes are packed with vitamin C and the greens are great for you, too. Bonus points if you've added one or two raw radishes, as well, because those enzymes can unlock the nutrients in the cooked radishes.

1/3 cup chicken stock or Upgraded Bone Broth (page 147)

2 tablespoons grass-fed unsalted butter

1 bunch radishes (12 ounces) with their greens, greens cleaned and radishes quartered

1 scallion, thinly sliced

2 teaspoons apple cider vinegar

Sea salt

In a medium saucepan, bring the stock and 1 tablespoon of the butter to a simmer over medium heat. Add the radishes and cook, stirring occasionally, until tender, about 6 minutes. Remove the pan from heat and stir in the remaining 1 tablespoon butter. Add the radish greens and scallion to the pan, return to low heat, and wilt the greens until just tender, about 2 minutes. Season with the vinegar and sea salt to taste.

RUTABAGA AND CELERY ROOT PUREE

SERVES 2

If you don't know what rutabaga is or think it's a medieval instrument, you'll discover a tasty new option with only moderate starch that you can enjoy. I love this with the Duck Confit (page 98) and the leftovers also pair well with the Braised Radishes and Greens (page 115) for a healthy lunch.

1   large rutabaga, peeled and cut into $\frac{1}{2}$-inch pieces

3   cups water

1   celery root, peeled and cut into $\frac{1}{2}$-inch pieces

3   tablespoons grass-fed unsalted butter

1   tablespoon high-quality olive oil

    Sea salt

In a medium saucepan fitted with a steamer insert, bring 2 cups water to a simmer over medium heat. Add the rutabaga, cover, and steam for 10 minutes. Add the remaining 1 cup water and the celery root, and steam for 20 minutes longer, until both vegetables are tender.

Transfer the vegetables to a food processor or blender. Add $\frac{1}{2}$ to $\frac{3}{4}$ cup of the steaming liquid (or water), the butter, and olive oil and puree. Season with salt to taste. Serve warm.

CAULIFLOWER "COUSCOUS"

SERVES 2

You're going to love cauliflower on the Bulletproof diet, especially after you try this recipe. It's such a great stand-in for couscous when prepared right, and the combination of butter and turmeric gives it just the right color and kick.

1	small head cauliflower (1¼ pounds), cut into 1-inch florets
1	teaspoon Bulletproof Brain Octane oil (or MCT or coconut oil)
2	tablespoons grass-fed unsalted butter
3	tablespoons water
¼	teaspoon ground turmeric
	Sea salt
1	tablespoon minced fresh chives

In a food processor, pulse the cauliflower until evenly broken into small couscous-size grains.

In a large skillet, combine the oil, butter, water, and turmeric and heat over medium heat until the butter melts. Add the cauliflower and cook, stirring often, until the cauliflower is tender and the liquid has evaporated, 6 to 7 minutes. Season with salt to taste and sprinkle with the chives.

BOK CHOY WITH CILANTRO-LIME BUTTER

SERVES 2

Both a leafy green and a cruciferous vegetable, bok choy acts as an ideal carrier for grass-fed butter. This recipe takes perfect advantage of that fact

$1\frac{1}{2}$ cups water

2   large heads bok choy, leaves separated

2   tablespoons Cilantro-Lime Compound Butter (page 201)

Sea salt

In a 6-quart pot fitted with a steamer insert, bring the water to a boil over medium heat. Add the bok choy and steam until just tender, about 7 minutes. Transfer the bok choy to a large bowl and toss with the compound butter and season with salt to taste.

SPICE-ROASTED FENNEL

SERVES 2

I used to think only foodies or hippies ate fennel, but I found that it has so much more flavor than celery. Today it's one of the dominant veggies in my garden with the best flavor. Try this at lunch with some smoked trout.

2	strips (2 inches long) orange zest
¾	teaspoon ground turmeric
1½	teaspoons fennel seeds
1	tablespoon fresh thyme leaves
1	tablespoon Bulletproof Brain Octane oil (or MCT or coconut oil)
1	tablespoon high-quality olive oil
	Sea salt
3	large fennel bulbs (2½ pounds total), trimmed (fronds minced and reserved for garnish), cored, and cut into ¼-inch-thick slices
4	teaspoons fresh lemon juice

Preheat the oven to 325°F. Line a baking sheet with parchment paper.

Very thinly sliver the orange zest. Place half of the orange zest in a large bowl and add the turmeric, fennel seeds, thyme, oils, and sea salt to taste. Add the sliced fennel, toss to coat, and spread out on the baking sheet. Bake, tossing once halfway through, until the fennel is tender, 35 to 40 minutes.

In a small bowl, combine the remaining orange zest, the lemon juice, and minced fennel fronds. Add to the baked fennel and toss to combine. Serve warm or at room temperature.

BEET AND AVOCADO TARTARE

SERVES 2

Beets can feed bacteria that release nitric oxide, which increases cardio vascular health. They are tasty, creamy and good for you. This dish is an easy side that pairs well with a simple Bulletproof fish, the Hanger Steak (page 93) or Perfect Parchment-Baked Salmon (page 77).

1	small bunch (3 or 4) golden beets, trimmed and washed
¾	cup water
1	lemon, divided into segments (see How to Segment Citrus, page 85), plus 1 tablespoon lemon juice
2	teaspoons high-quality olive oil
2	teaspoons Bulletproof Brain Octane oil (or MCT or coconut oil)
2	tablespoons minced fresh herbs (such as parsley, chives, and oregano)
	Sea salt
1	avocado, cut into ¼-inch dice
2	radishes, thinly sliced

Preheat the oven to 320°F.

In an 8 x 8-inch baking pan, combine the beets with the water, cover with foil, and bake until tender when pierced with a knife, 45 to 60 minutes. Let cool for about 30 minutes to a little over room temperature. Peel the beets, cut into ¼-inch dice, and place in a medium bowl.

In a small bowl, whisk together the lemon juice, oils, and herbs. Season with salt to taste.

Add the dressing to the beets along with the avocado, radishes, and lemon segments. Season with salt to taste and toss gently.

BRAISED CABBAGE

SERVES 2, WITH LEFTOVERS

This is actually a traditional meal throughout Europe and Russia. My wife is Swedish and had a Czezh influence growing up, so she was introduced to the concept early on. Enjoy this recipe with Ginger-Braised Ribs (page 92), Hanger Steak (page 93), or Pork Chops with Herbed Crust (page 95).

2	tablespoons grass-fed unsalted butter
1	small leek, well washed, white and light green parts only, cut into $\frac{1}{4}$-inch-thick slices (optional)
2	sprigs of rosemary
1	red cabbage ($1\frac{3}{4}$ pounds), shredded
$\frac{1}{2}$	cup apple cider vinegar
$\frac{3}{4}$	cup chicken stock or Upgraded Bone Broth (page 147)
	Sea salt
1	cup fresh cranberries
3 to 4	tablespoons raw honey (optional)

Preheat the oven to 300°F.

In a large ovenproof pot, melt the butter over medium-low heat. Add the leek (if using), rosemary, cabbage, vinegar, stock, and a pinch of sea salt and stir to combine. Cover, transfer to the oven, and bake for 15 minutes.

Stir in the cranberries, re-cover, and continue baking until the cabbage is tender and the cranberries burst, about 15 minutes longer. Stir in honey to taste (if using) and season with sea salt to taste.

CARROT AND CABBAGE SLAW

SERVES 2

Eating tons of raw cabbage can cause thyroid issues, but I'll admit that occasionally it is delicious. The trick is to finely slice your cabbage. In general, you want it lightly cooked because heat reduces oxalates. Here, however, the lemon juice neutralizes the oxalates instead.

½	small head red cabbage, finely sliced
2	teaspoons fresh lemon juice
1½	teaspoons coarse sea salt
1	pound carrots, grated
1	scallion, quartered crosswise and thinly sliced lengthwise
2	radishes, thinly sliced
2	tablespoons plus 1 teaspoon apple cider vinegar
1 to 2	tablespoons Bulletproof Brain Octane oil (or MCT or coconut oil) (to taste)
5	basil leaves, thinly sliced

In a large bowl, combine the cabbage, lemon juice, and coarse salt. Let stand for 15 minutes. Drain the cabbage of any liquid. Add the carrots, scallion, radishes, vinegar, oil, and basil and toss to combine. Adjust the seasonings to taste.

STEAMED ARTICHOKES
WITH SALMON AND VINAIGRETTE

SERVES 2

Having lived in Silicon Valley near the artichoke capital, I've eaten thousands, but I know many people who have never had one. They are not very difficult to prepare, and the rewards are worth your effort.

Juice of 1 large lemon

2 large globe artichokes (about ¾ pound each)

2 teaspoons apple cider vinegar

1½ tablespoons Bulletproof Brain Octane oil (or MCT or coconut oil)

1 tablespoon high-quality olive oil

1 tablespoon chopped fresh parsley

1 tablespoon capers, chopped

Sea salt

8 ounces smoked salmon

Fill a large bowl with water. Measure out and set aside 2 tablespoons lemon juice and add the remaining juice to the bowl of water. Trim the artichoke stems and peel them. Cut 1 inch off the tops. Remove the outer leaves and submerge the artichokes in the lemon water (leave them submerged while working).

In a large pot fitted with a steamer insert, bring 3 cups water to a simmer over medium heat. Add the artichokes, cover, and steam until the leaves are tender and pull away easily, 30 to 35 minutes, flipping the artichokes over halfway through.

Meanwhile, in a small bowl, combine the reserved 2 tablespoons lemon juice, the vinegar, oils, parsley, and capers. Season with salt to taste. Set the vinaigrette aside.

Transfer the artichokes to a cutting board and let cool, about 10 minutes. When the artichokes are cool enough to handle, halve them lengthwise and spoon out and discard the fibrous bristles above the heart choke.

Serve the artichoke halves topped with a few slices of salmon and drizzled with vinaigrette. Pull off the artichoke leaves and eat them first, then cut up the heart to enjoy with the salmon.

BUTTERED BRUSSELS SPROUTS

SERVES 2

As a kid, I hated sprouts—like many people! They were mushy and stinky. But when you learn to cook them right, they're amazing, especially in butter. Please don't blacken the outside as so many restaurants do. It may taste good, but it's not good for you. Brussels sprouts are chock-full of vitamin C, folate, potassium, calcium, and fiber.

1 pound Brussels sprouts, trimmed

2 tablespoons grass-fed unsalted butter, at room temperature

Finely grated zest of 1 lemon

Pinch of cayenne pepper (optional)

Sea salt

In a medium pot fitted with a steamer insert, bring 2½ cups water to a boil over medium heat. Add the Brussels sprouts and steam until tender, 8 to 10 minutes. Transfer to a medium bowl and toss with the butter, lemon zest, and cayenne pepper (if using.) Season with salt to taste.

BUTTERED KALE

SERVES 2

Let's face it: No one likes raw kale. Kale prepared this way is better tasting than raw and it's better for you as well.

1 tablespoon ghee

1 tablespoon water

1 bunch (12 ounces) lacinato kale, thick stems and ribs removed, torn into 3-inch pieces

2 tablespoons grass-fed unsalted butter

1 tablespoon chopped fresh dill

   Sea salt

   Lemon juice

In a large, deep skillet or Dutch oven, heat the ghee and water over medium heat. Add the kale, cover, and cook, stirring often, until just wilted, about 3 minutes. Add the butter and stir until the butter melts and coats the kale, about 1 minute longer. Remove from the heat and stir in the dill and salt and the lemon juice to taste. Serve hot.

BUTTERNUT SQUASH

SERVES 2

If you haven't tried butternut squash, now's the time. It's a reasonable carb and is high in vitamins. I'm growing dozens of them as I write this. This recipe makes a great side when you're in maintenance mode—not protein fasting or intermittent fasting.

1   lemon, halved

1   butternut squash (2 pounds), peeled, seeded, and cut into ½-inch chunks

1   tablespoon Bulletproof Brain Octane oil (or MCT or coconut oil)

1   tablespoon ghee, melted

2   teaspoons minced fresh herbs (such as rosemary, oregano, and sage)

Sea salt

Preheat the oven to 325°F. Line a large baking sheet with parchment paper.

Cut one of the lemon halves into ¼-inch-thick slices. Set the other lemon half aside.

In a large bowl, combine the lemon slices, squash, oil, ghee, herbs, and salt to taste and toss to combine. Spread the squash out on the baking sheet. Bake until tender, tossing once halfway through, 40 to 45 minutes. Squeeze the reserved lemon half over the squash.

CARROT AND SWEET POTATO MASH

SERVES 2

When I make this dish, I like to add some Bulletproof Brain Octane oil so I don't feel hungry. It also delivers extra brain-boosting fat and satisfying flavor.

1½ cups water

1 bunch carrots, cut into 1-inch pieces

2 sweet potatoes, peeled and cut into 1-inch pieces

2 tablespoons grass-fed unsalted butter

Sea salt

In a medium saucepan, bring the water to a simmer over medium-high heat. Add the carrots and sweet potatoes, cover, and cook until tender, about 8 minutes. Transfer the vegetables to a blender and process with ½ cup of the cooking liquid and the butter. Season with salt to taste.

COLLARDS AND BACON

SERVES 2

It used to be common to use bacon as flavoring, but then it fell out of style. Today, bacon is back. It has great flavor, and scientists have recently discovered that you have fat receptors that love this taste. Collards, like other cruciferous vegetables, need to be cooked to reduce their oxalates, but cooking too long diminishes their nutrient content. This short "braise" with bacon retains nutrients and packs flavor.

2	slices pastured bacon, cut into $1/2$-inch pieces
1	bunch collard greens (12 ounces), tough ribs removed, leaves cut into 1-inch pieces
1	cup chicken stock or Upgraded Bone Broth (page 147)
1	small leek, white and light green parts only, cut into $1/2$-inch pieces
1	tablespoon grass-fed unsalted butter
2 to 3	teaspoons apple cider vinegar (to taste)
	Sea salt

In a medium pot, cook the bacon over medium-low heat until golden but not crisp, about 8 minutes. Add the collards and chicken stock and cook, stirring occasionally, for 8 minutes. Add the leek and cook until the collards are just tender, about 4 minutes longer. Stir in the butter and vinegar and season with sea salt to taste.

LOW-ROASTED BROCCOLI RABE

SERVES 2

The first time I saw it, I thought broccoli rabe was young broccoli, but I'm told it's called rabe. All I know is, it tastes great. And this preparation showcases the flavor while keeping the nutrients intact.

1   bunch broccoli rabe (1 pound), trimmed

1   tablespoon Bulletproof Brain Octane oil (or MCT or coconut oil)

2   tablespoons ghee, melted

2   scallions, cut into 1/2-inch pieces, white and greens kept separate

3   tablespoons water

    Sea salt

Preheat the oven to 325°F.

In a large bowl, combine broccoli rabe, oil, ghee, scallion whites, water, and sea salt to taste and toss to coat. Transfer to a 9 x 13-inch baking pan and bake, uncovered, turning at 8-minute intervals, until the broccoli rabe is tender, 22 to 24 minutes. Season with salt to taste and serve sprinkled with the scallion greens.

BROCCOLI WITH TAPENADE AND BACON

SERVES 2

I believe Mother Nature engineered broccoli to hold an incredible amount of nutrients in all those little green folded nooks. And when you add bacon and olives, this becomes a perfect food source. Remember to cook the broccoli until it's just tender, to keep oxalates low and vitamins C and K intact.

- 1 head broccoli (1 pound), trimmed and cut into florets
- 2 slices of pastured, preservative-free bacon, cut into $\frac{1}{4}$-inch pieces ($2\frac{1}{2}$ ounces)
- 2 tablespoons Tapenade (page 204)
- 2 teaspoons apple cider vinegar
- 1 tablespoon ground whole raw almonds (optional)

Place a steamer basket in a 6-quart pot with a lid and add $1\frac{1}{2}$ cups water. Cover and bring the water to a boil over medium-high heat. Add the broccoli and steam until just tender, about 8 minutes.

In a large, high-sided skillet, cook the bacon over medium-low heat until firm but not crisp, about 6 minutes. Take off the heat and add the tapenade and cider vinegar, whisking to combine. Add the broccoli and stir to combine. Top with almonds (if using) and serve.

ARTICHOKES WITH DILL AND MINT

SERVES 2

Don't toss those artichoke leaves. They have delicious flesh you can scrape off with your teeth. Dip the leaves in melted grass-fed butter, Bulletproof Brain Octane oil, or melted Cilantro-Lime Butter (page 201) for a tasty treat. Serve this herbed preparation with Perfect Parchment-Baked Salmon (page 77).

- 3 tablespoons fresh lemon juice
- 4 globe artichokes (about ¾ pound each)
- 3 tablespoons high-quality olive oil
- 2 teaspoons Bulletproof Brain Octane oil (or MCT or coconut oil)
- Coarse sea salt
- 1 small scallion, thinly sliced
- 1 tablespoon coarsely chopped fresh dill
- 2 or 3 teaspoons mint leaves, torn

Fill a large bowl with water and add half the lemon juice. Trim 1 inch off the artichoke stems and tops and peel the stems. Holding the artichokes submerged in the lemon water, remove the tough outer leaves.

In a large pot fitted with a steamer insert, bring 4 cups water to a simmer over medium heat. Add the artichokes, cover, and steam until the artichokes are tender when pierced with a knife and the leaves are tender and pull out easily, about 1 hour and 15 minutes (add more hot water as needed).

Transfer the artichokes to a cutting board to cool slightly. When cool enough to handle, pull off all the leaves. Use a spoon to scoop out the fibrous bristles, discarding them, so that the heart and stem remain. Cut the heart and stem into ¼-inch pieces.

In a small bowl, whisk together the remaining 1½ tablespoons lemon juice, 1½ tablespoons of the olive oil, the Brain Octane oil, and sea salt to taste. Stir in the artichokes, scallion, dill, and mint, turning to coat. Drizzle with the remaining 1½ tablespoons olive oil.

ASPARAGUS IN GINGER BROTH

SERVES 2

This side also makes a great soup: Puree the cooked asparagus and broth in a blender, adding 1 or 2 tablespoons of water if needed. Drizzle with olive oil or Bulletproof Brain Octane oil.

1 cup chicken stock or Upgraded Bone Broth (page 147)

1 tablespoon thinly sliced peeled fresh ginger

1 piece (3-inch) lemongrass, split

1 pound asparagus, trimmed, peeled if the stalks are large

1 teaspoon Bulletproof Brain Octane oil (or MCT or coconut oil)

Sea salt

1 scallion, halved lengthwise and cut into 3-inch lengths

2 tablespoons grass-fed unsalted butter

Pinch of cayenne powder (optional)

1 teaspoon fresh lemon juice

In a medium saucepan, combine the stock, ginger, and lemongrass and bring to a simmer over medium heat. Cook for 2 minutes to develop flavors.

Add the asparagus, Brain Octane oil, and a pinch of sea salt. Stir, cover, and steam for 2 minutes. Add the scallion and cook until the asparagus is tender, 1 minute more. With a slotted spoon, transfer the asparagus and scallion to a bowl. Discard the lemongrass and whisk the butter and cayenne (if using) into the broth. Season with the lemon juice and sea salt to taste. Pour the broth over the asparagus and serve.

BACON-WILTED ESCAROLE

SERVES 2

Escarole is another one of those vegetables I didn't know much about, but now that I play around with different kinds of greens, I've found it to be a tasty and versatile addition to many recipes. It's also great in soups.

1 tablespoon Bulletproof Brain Octane oil (or MCT or coconut oil)

1 thick slice (1 ounce) slab pastured bacon, cut into ¼-inch pieces

1 head escarole, washed and torn into 2-inch-long pieces

1½ teaspoons grated lemon zest

1½ teaspoons apple cider vinegar

Coarse sea salt

2 tablespoons chopped walnuts (optional)

1 teaspoon fresh oregano leaves

In a large skillet, combine the Brain Octane oil and bacon. Cook over medium heat until the bacon is almost crisp and cooked, but not burnt, about 3 minutes. Add the escarole and lemon zest and cook, turning often, until just wilted, about 3 minutes. Add the vinegar and cook until tender, 1 minute more. Season to taste with sea salt. Serve topped top with walnuts (if using) and oregano.

BRAISED ROMAINE AND ENDIVE

SERVES 2

Warm lettuce? Sure! This is a great Bulletproof side for lots of dishes; it's especially good with the Duck Confit (page 98).

1	tablespoon Bulletproof Brain Octane oil (or MCT or coconut oil)
1	Belgian endive, trimmed, cored, and cut lengthwise into eighths
2	tablespoons chopped leek, white part only
1	teaspoon grated lemon zest
1	head romaine lettuce, trimmed, washed, and leaves separated
¼	cup Upgraded Bone Broth (page 147) or chicken stock
	Coarse sea salt
⅛	teaspoon ground turmeric
3	tablespoons cold grass-fed unsalted butter
	Lemon wedges, for serving

Heat a large skillet over medium heat. Add the Brain Octane oil and endive. Cook, reducing the heat to medium-low and turning occasionally until the endive is just starting to wilt, about 3 minutes. Add the leek, lemon zest, and lettuce and cook, turning to coat the lettuce in the lemon zest, about 1 minute. Add the broth and a pinch of sea salt and cook, stirring, until the endive and lettuce are crisp-tender, about 4 minutes.

Transfer the greens to a plate, leaving the liquid in the pan. Remove the pan from the heat and whisk in the turmeric, then the butter, 1 tablespoon at a time. Pour the sauce over the greens. Season with sea salt to taste and serve with lemon wedges.

CUCUMBER AND AVOCADO

SERVES 2

Once in maintenance mode, if you require protein at breakfast, try this "salad" to get you started; it has a great combination of protein and fat, and a good serving of potassium, too.

- 1 large pastured egg yolk
- 1 teaspoon grated lime zesl
- 1 tablespoon plus 2 teaspoons fresh lime juice
- 1 tablespoon water
- ³⁄₄ teaspoon grated fresh ginger
- ¹⁄₂ teaspoon coarse sea salt
- ¹⁄₄ teaspoon high-quality red pepper flakes (optional)
- 2 tablespoons high-quality olive oil
- 1 tablespoon Bulletproof Brain Octane oil (or MCT or coconut oil)
- 1 large cucumber, peeled, halved, and seeded
- 1 scallion, dark green tops only, minced
- 1 avocado, pitted, peeled, and cut into ¹⁄₄-inch dice
- ¹⁄₄ cup fresh cilantro leaves

In a large bowl, whisk together the egg yolk, lime zest, lime juice, water, ginger, sea salt, and red pepper flakes (if using). Whisking constantly, drizzle in the oils until you have an emulsified dressing.

Cut the cucumber lengthwise into eighths, then crosswise into ¹⁄₂-inch cubes and add to the bowl. Stir in the scallion and avocado and toss well to coat. Adjust the seasoning to taste and top with the cilantro.

KALE CARBONARA

SERVES 2

The eggs here enrich the sauce and keep all their micronutrients intact thanks to minimal heating. Be sure your eggs are pastured, or you risk not benefiting from their powerhouse of vitamins (A and E) and nutrients (omega-3s).

2 large pastured egg yolks, beaten

2 tablespoons coconut cream (from the top of an unshaken can of coconut milk)

4 teaspoons Bulletproof Brain Octane oil (or MCT or coconut oil)

2 slices regular-cut pastured bacon, cut into ¼-inch pieces

1 scallion, white part only, thinly sliced (optional)

1 bunch lacinato kale, center ribs removed, finely sliced

Sea salt

Lemon wedges, for serving

In a small bowl, whisk together the egg yolks and coconut cream.

In a large skillet, combine the Brain Octane oil and bacon and cook over medium heat for 2 minutes. Add the scallion (if using) and cook, stirring, until the bacon is cooked and the scallion tender, 1 minute more.

Add the kale to the pan and cook, stirring often, until just tender and most of the liquid has evaporated, about 3 minutes. Reduce the heat to low and add the yolk-coconut mixture, stirring often to coat. Be careful not to overcook the eggs. Season with sea salt and serve with a squeeze of lemon.

SWISS CHARD WITH FENNEL SALT

SERVES 2

The Bulletproof Fennel Salt adds just the kick to this Bulletproof green. Organic chard from a farmers' market and some Brain Octane and olive oil plus lemon juice are all you need to put together this quick, flavor- and nutrient-packed Bulletproof side.

2	teaspoons Bulletproof Brain Octane oil (or MCT or coconut oil)
1	bunch Swiss chard, thick stems removed, leaves torn
1/8	teaspoon Fennel Salt (page 200), or to taste
1	teaspoon high-quality olive oil
1/2	teaspoon fresh lemon juice

Heat a large skillet over medium heat for about 2 minutes. Add the Brain Octane oil, Swiss chard, and fennel salt. Cook, stirring often, until the chard is wilted and tender, about 3 minutes. Transfer to a plate and drizzle with the olive oil and lemon juice.

TURNIP GRATIN

SERVES 2

When you've got a craving for something really carby like mac & cheese, try this as a smart stand-in. Turnips are high in vitamin C, and this pairs beautifully with the Bulletproof Chicken (page 104).

3	tablespoons grass-fed unsalted butter, plus more for the baking dish
1½	cups canned coconut milk, well shaken
½	large leek, white and light green parts only, split lengthwise and cut crosswise into ¼-inch pieces
2	teaspoons fresh thyme leaves, coarsely chopped
	Coarse sea salt
3	medium turnips, peeled and cut into ¼-inch-thick wedges
1	tablespoon fresh oregano leaves or minced chives, for serving

Preheat the oven to 350°F. Butter an 8 x 8-inch (2-quart) baking dish.

In a small saucepan, combine the coconut milk, leek, thyme, and 1 teaspoon coarse sea salt. Bring to a simmer and cook until the leek is soft, 5 to 6 minutes.

Make a single layer with about half of the turnips in the buttered baking dish, overlapping and aligning them as best you can to make a single flat layer. Pour half of the coconut-mixture over the turnips. Dollop with 1½ tablespoons of the butter. Repeat layering with the remaining turnips, tucking in small pieces as needed. Pour the remaining coconut milk mixture over the turnips and dot with remaining 1½ tablespoons butter.

Cover with foil and place on a rimmed baking sheet. Bake until the turnips are tender, about 1 hour. Uncover and bake until the cream is reduced, about 15 minutes. Serve sprinkled with oregano or chives.

ZUCCHINI WITH PESTO

SERVES 2

Zucchini is at its peak in the summertime, where it is best purchased locally from a farmers' market (GMO zucchini is unfortunately common).

2 or 3	zucchini (or a combination of zucchini and summer squash), cut into $1/4$-inch slices
$1/4$	cup whole raw almonds
$1/2$	cup fresh parsley leaves, washed
1	bunch basil, leaves picked, plus 3 or 4 leaves reserved and torn for serving
1	tablespoon minced fresh chives
1	teaspoon coarse sea salt
2	tablespoons Bulletproof Brain Octane oil (or MCT or coconut oil)
$1/2$	cup high-quality olive oil
2	tablespoons fresh lemon juice

In a medium pot fitted with a steamer insert, bring 2 cups of water to a simmer over medium heat. Add the zucchini and steam until crisp-tender, 6 to 8 minutes. Set aside to cool.

Meanwhile, in a food processor, pulse the almonds to a fine meal. Add the parsley, basil, chives, and sea salt and pulse to combine. With the processor running, add the oils in a slow stream until well combined. Measure out $1/4$ cup of the pesto (reserve the remainder for another use) and stir in the lemon juice.

Layer the zucchini on a plate with the reserved basil leaves. Drizzle the pesto sauce over the zucchini and season to taste with sea salt.

CHOCOLATE-DRIZZLED PEAR SALAD WITH LEMON-ROSEMARY VINAIGRETTE

SERVES 2

This delicious salad isn't a dessert, even though antioxidant-rich chocolate is an ingredient. Instead, I recommend this for festive meals, like Thanksgiving, since it's sure to impress guests. Doubling or even quadrupling the quantity for a crowd is fine.

Lemon-Rosemary Vinaigrette

Juice of $1/2$ lemon

$1/2$ cup coconut oil or Bulletproof Brain Octane oil (or MCT or coconut oil)

1 garlic clove, smashed

1 tablespoon fresh rosemary, chopped

$1/8$ teaspoon Dijon mustard

1 thick slice of pear (about $1\frac{1}{4}$ inches), peeled

Pinch of Himalayan pink salt

Freshly ground pepper

Salad

3 cups mixed baby greens

1 small shallot, sliced

1 pear, unpeeled and sliced

1 teaspoon raw honey

1 tablespoon chopped fresh thyme

$1/2$ ounce bittersweet or 70 percent cacao chocolate

1 to 2 pinches of cayenne pepper (to taste)

$1/4$ teaspoon finely chopped fresh rosemary

$1/4$ cup crumbled goat cheese

Preheat the oven to 350°F. Line a baking sheet with parchment paper.

For the vinaigrette: In a blender, combine all the ingredients and blend until smooth. Set aside.

For the salad: In a large bowl, combine the baby greens and shallot and set aside.

Arrange the pear slices on the baking sheet and drizzle lightly with the honey and sprinkle with the thyme. Bake until just soft, 8 to 10 minutes.

Meanwhile, in a small bowl set over a small saucepan of simmering water, melt the chocolate. Stir in the cayenne and rosemary and let sit.

When the pears are done, remove from the oven. To serve, toss the greens with the vinaigrette and divide between 2 salad plates. Top with the pears and crumbled goat cheese. Using a spoon, drizzle the pears lightly with the melted chocolate.

CAULIFLOWER-BACON MASH

SERVES 2 TO 4

You will never miss eating mashed potatoes now that you can have deliciously creamy, bacon-flavored mashed cauliflower instead!

½	pound pastured, uncured bacon, diced
¾ to 1	large head cauliflower, cut into florets
4	tablespoons grass-fed unsalted butter
2	tablespoons Bulletproof Brain Octane oil (or MCT or coconut oil)
½	tablespoon apple cider vinegar
	Sea salt

In a large skillet, lightly cook the bacon over medium-low heat. Do not let it get crispy (keep those fats intact) and do not let the fat smoke. Set the bacon aside and reserve the fat in the pan.

In a pot fitted with a steamer insert, bring water to a boil. Add the cauliflower, cover, and steam until tender, 15 to 20 minutes.

In a high-powered blender, blend three-fourths of the cauliflower with the butter, oil, vinegar, and salt to taste. Stir in the bacon and remaining cauliflower. Pulse the mixture until chunky. For amazing flavor, add 1 to 2 tablespoons of the bacon fat (as long as it didn't smoke when you were cooking the bacon at a low temperature).

LOW-CARB RICE WITH HONEY

SERVES 4 TO 6

Recent research has found that cooking white rice with coconut oil and cooling it immediately after produces rice with resistant starch, which doesn't cause a spike in blood sugar levels. Instead, resistant starch may improve insulin sensitivity, enhance sleep quality, and increase energy levels and mental clarity. This could be a great dessert for protein-fasting days, when you want to enjoy a few more carbs but still stay Bulletproof.

1½ cups water

1 cup sushi rice

3 tablespoons Bulletproof Brain Octane oil (or MCT or coconut oil), plus more for serving

2 tablespoons grass-fed unsalted butter, melted

1 teaspoon raw honey

Pinch of Himalayan pink salt

In a small saucepan, bring the water to a boil.

Meanwhile, rinse the rice well in cold water and drain.

Add the rinsed rice and Brain Octane oil to the boiling water and reduce the heat to low. Cover and cook until tender, about 20 minutes.

Remove the rice from the heat and immediately transfer to an ovenproof casserole or a baking sheet. Place in the fridge to cool for at least 1 hour. You can spread the rice out in a flat layer or split it into thumb-sized portions (think nigiri sushi) on the sheet or in the casserole before putting it in the fridge so that it cools more quickly.

When the rice is almost cool, preheat the oven to warm.

Place the rice in the oven to warm through. Drizzle the butter, honey, salt, and—if you like—more Brain Octane oil over the rice and serve.

CHAPTER 7

SOUPS AND BROTHS

The first thing to talk about when we think of soups is bone broth, usually known as stock. If you're not yet familiar with bone broths, you're in for a supernutritious Bulletproof treat. These soups, long the centerpiece of Traditional Chinese Medicine and Ayurveda, are some of the healthiest meals you can make. Created by slowly simmering high-quality meat bones over low heat for an extended time, bone broths use a gentle cooking method to extract rich marrow and collagen from the bones, delivering a superboost of nutrients for all kinds of benefits to your system, from cellular repair to heightened immunity.

While bone broths do have to cook for a long time, they're really just a matter of easy assembly—and careful sourcing, of course. It's one of those dishes that falls under the old "set it and forget it" approach. You do have to be very careful about the quality of the bones, checking the provenance, but that won't surprise you by now. Because the technique is so effective at extracting every last drop of nutritional value from the bones, you must imagine that if the bones were of low quality, the process would likewise suck out every last toxin. So please, if you're going to make bone broths—and you should—remember that it needs to be done properly. It would be better to not do it at all than to make one with an inferior-quality product, which would just serve to give you a super-dose of toxicity. Once you've mastered the not-very-difficult process of making bone broth, you can make an infinite number of varieties, blending in seasonings you prefer like cumin or ginger (though you should see my notes on spices and remember that ginger, when paired with fats, can turn bitter).

I recommend making bone broth once a week or a couple of times a month and just having it on hand as a great, warming cup of nutrients whenever you like. The flavor is rich and robust, but it has a thin, elegant texture, so you could even serve it to guests in a demitasse cup as an amuse-bouche instead of consommé.

Warming liquids don't have to be broths, of course; they can be thicker and even creamy. When I'm making a warm soup that's *not* a bone broth, sometimes I'll blend in nuts to give it a rich, creamy consistency. Take my Cauliflower and Cashew Soup (page 151): It really simulates a creamy texture. Between the nuts and the butter, you won't miss any of the heavy cream that's usually associated with velvety soups.

People are accustomed to warm soups and cold smoothies, but it doesn't have to be that way. My Chilled Avocado and Cucumber Soup (page 152) is perfect chilled on a summer day, or as an elegant starter to a light meal. I even made a Cold Lettuce Soup (page 153), which sounds fantastically bland, but you're going to be amazed by the flavor profiles. There are so many exciting greens now to choose from compared to 15 years ago when it was only iceberg and romaine. As with temperature change-ups, Bulletproof soups can be sweet, and smoothies can be savory (see my exciting change-ups on smoothies in Chapter 8, starting on page 170.) If you open your mind to what food types "belong" in what categories, you'll double the options you have for staying Bulletproof, 24/7.

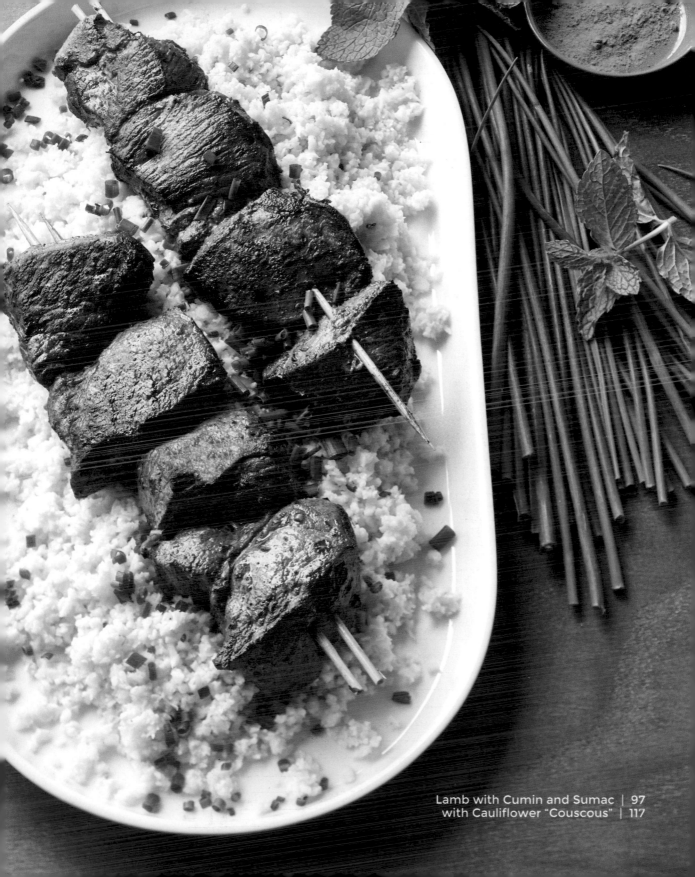

Lamb with Cumin and Sumac | 97
with Cauliflower "Couscous" | 117

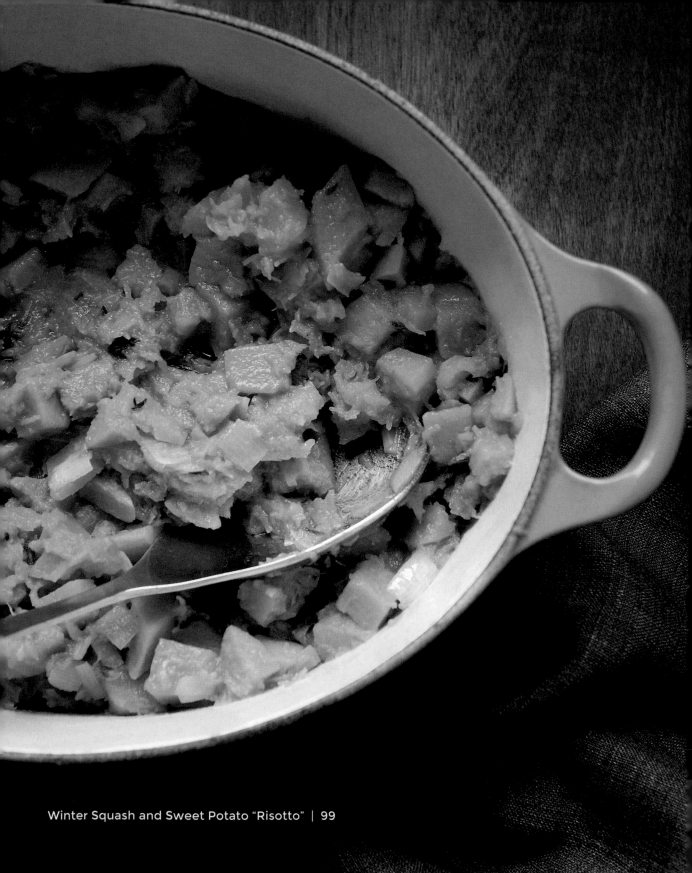

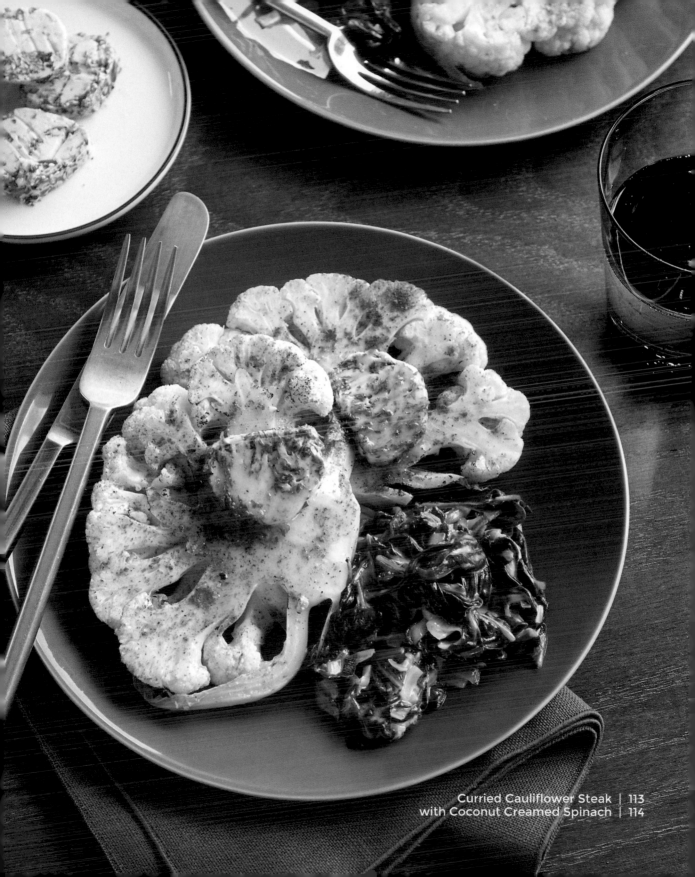

Curried Cauliflower Steak | 113
with Coconut Creamed Spinach | 114

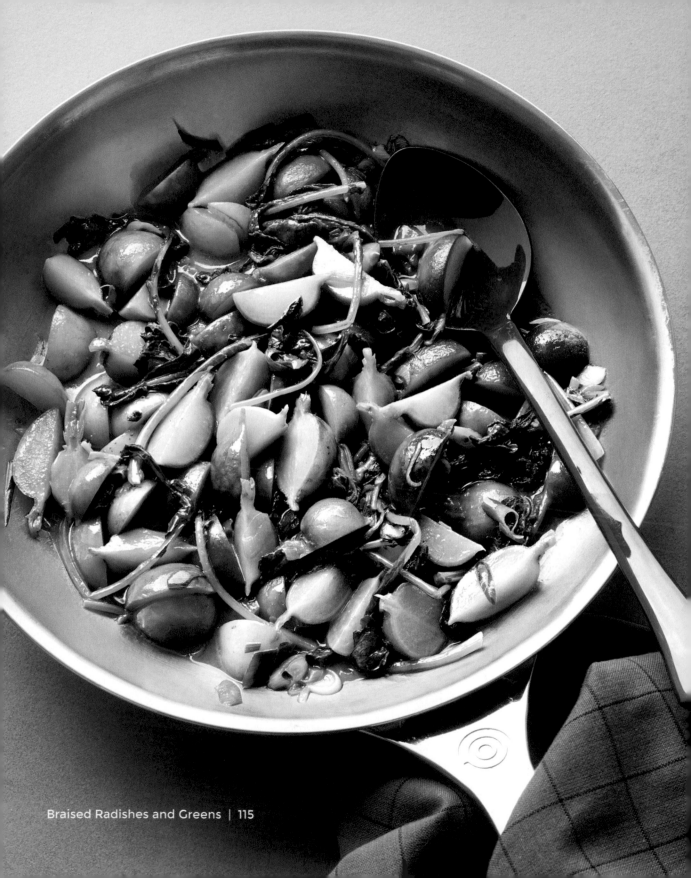

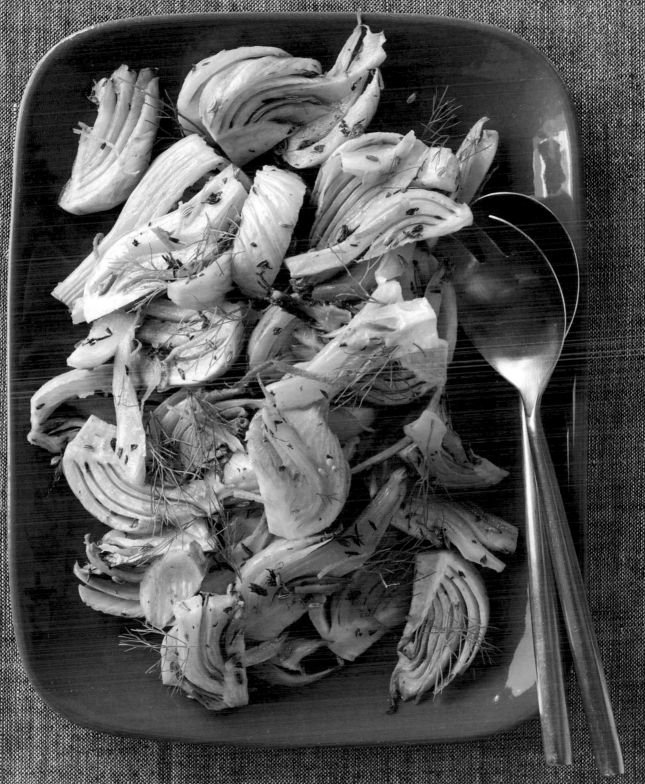

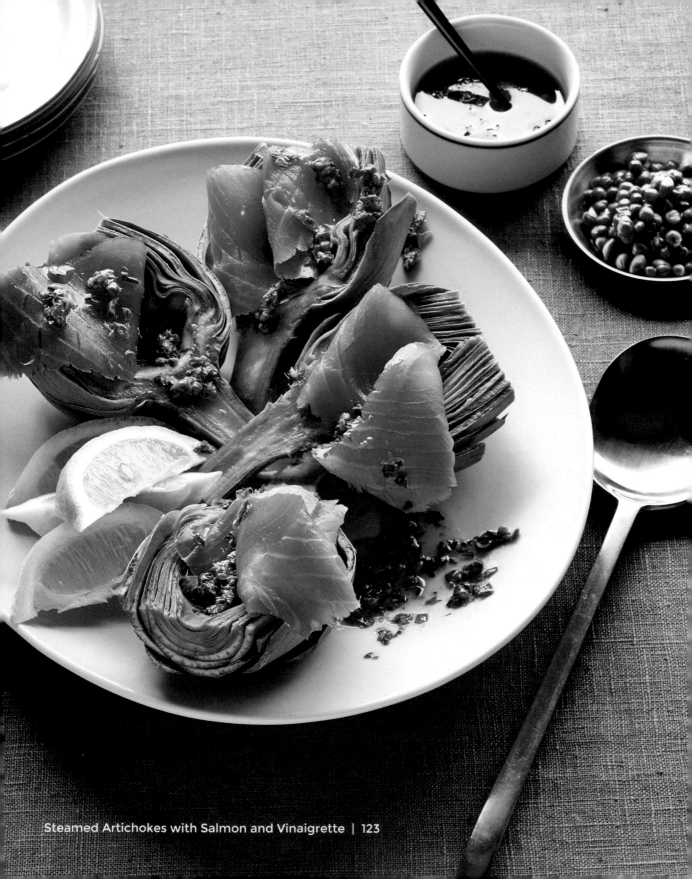

Steamed Artichokes with Salmon and Vinaigrette | 123

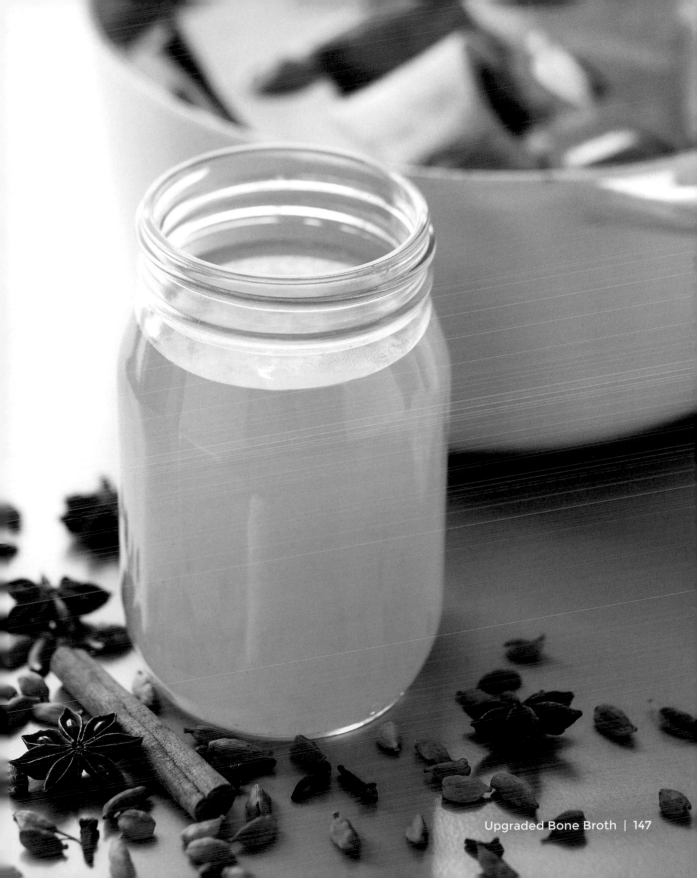

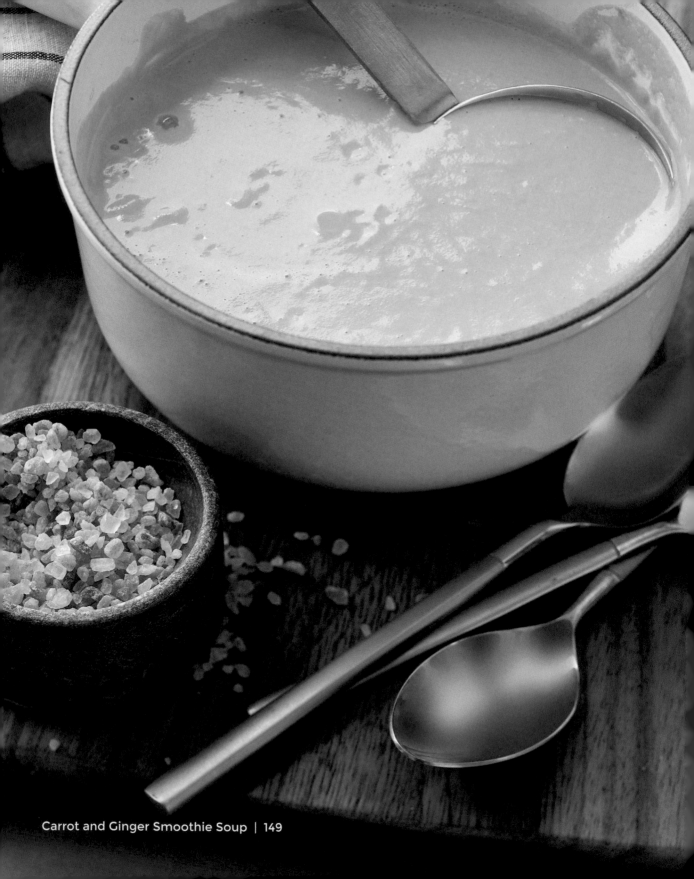

Carrot and Ginger Smoothie Soup | 149

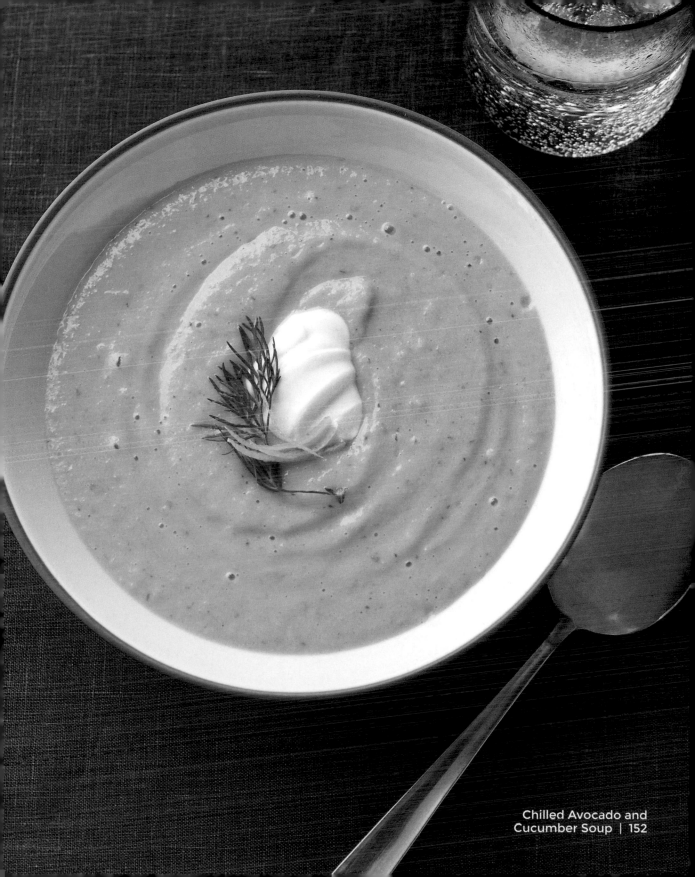

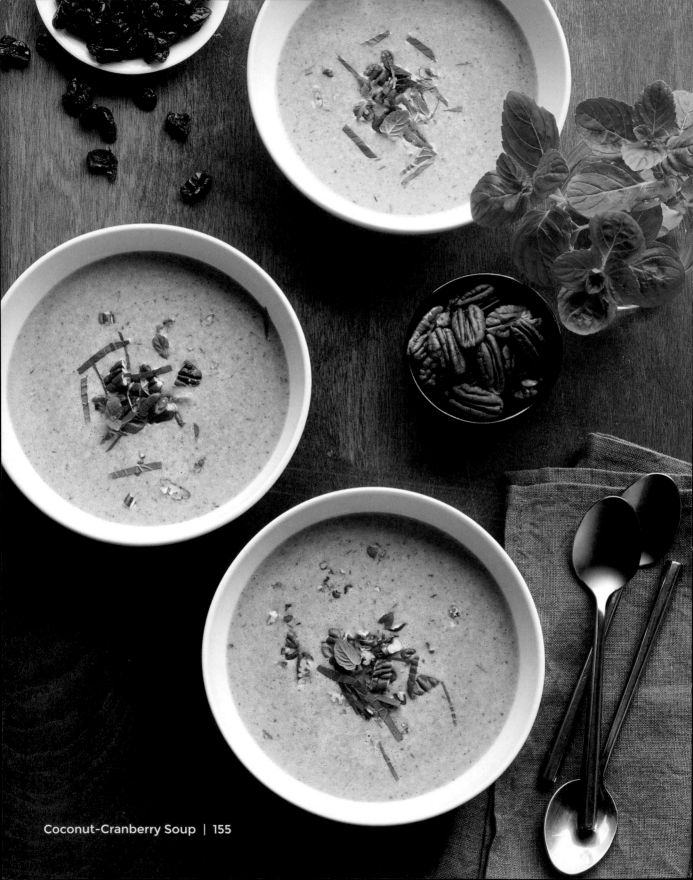

Coconut-Cranberry Soup | 155

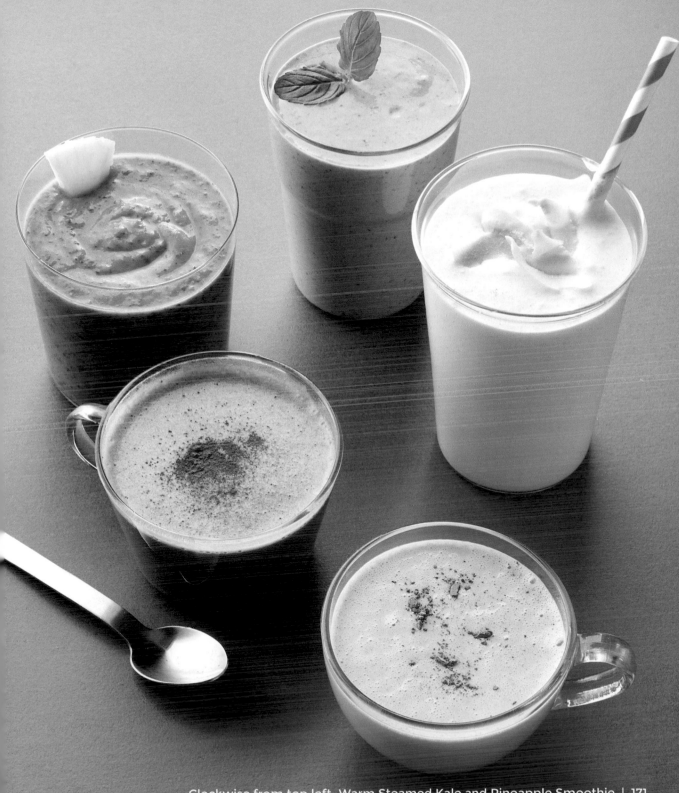

Clockwise from top left: Warm Steamed Kale and Pineapple Smoothie | 171,
Strawberries and Cream Smoothie | 173, Coconut Smoothie | 172,
Green Tea Latte | 169, Bulletproof Coconut Hot Chocolate | 168

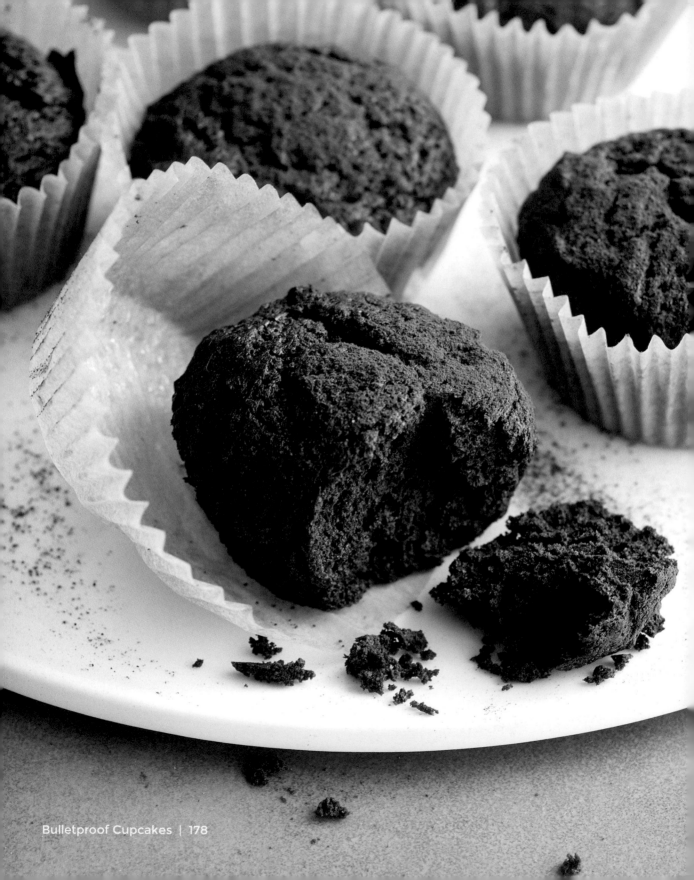

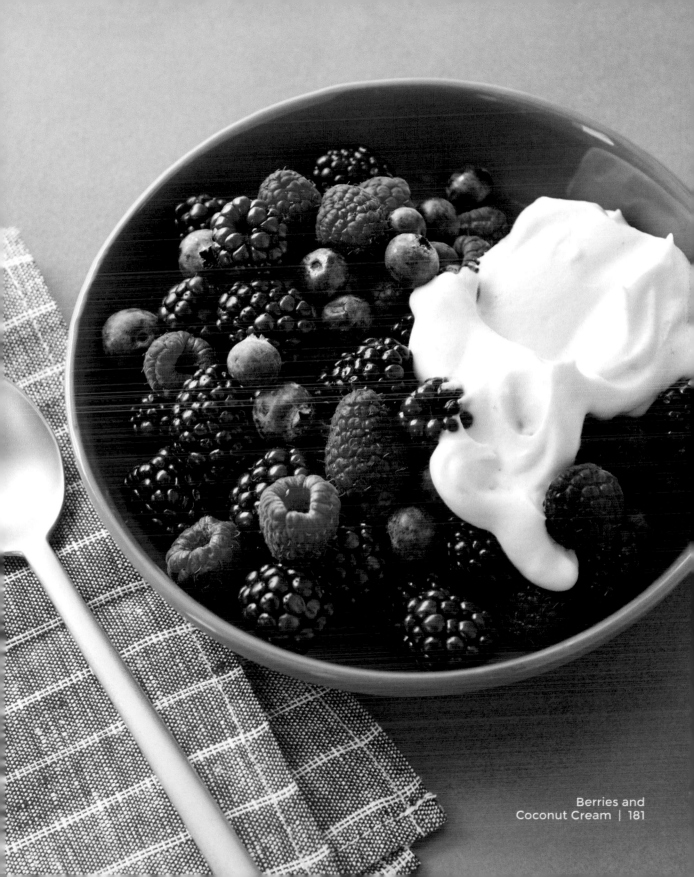

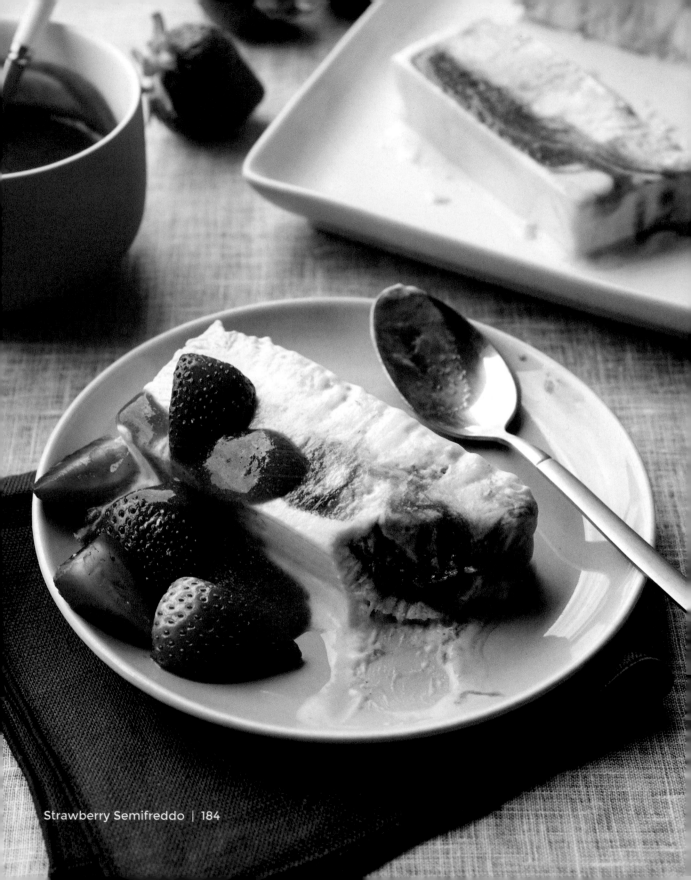

Strawberry Semifreddo | 184

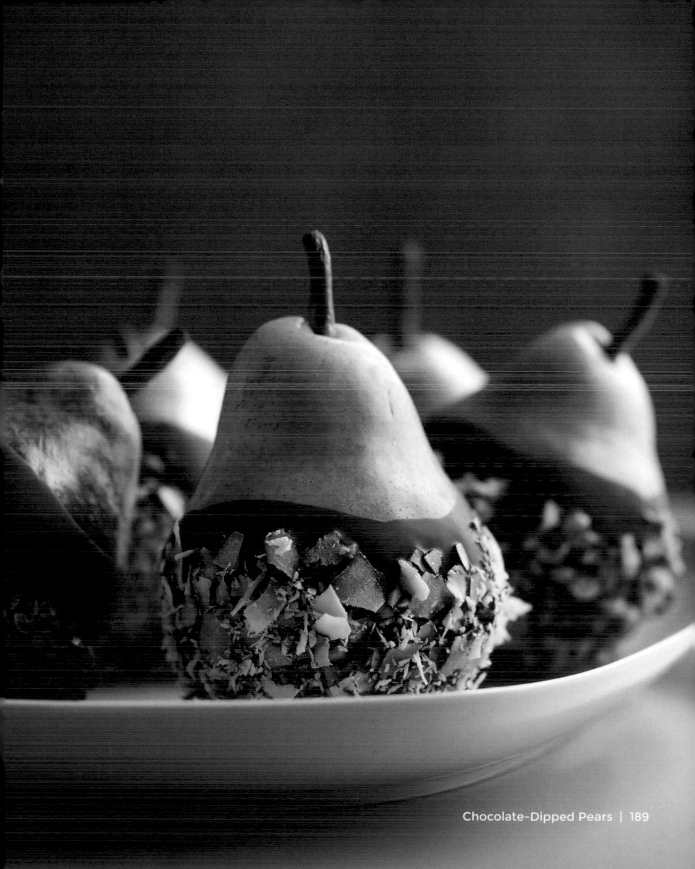

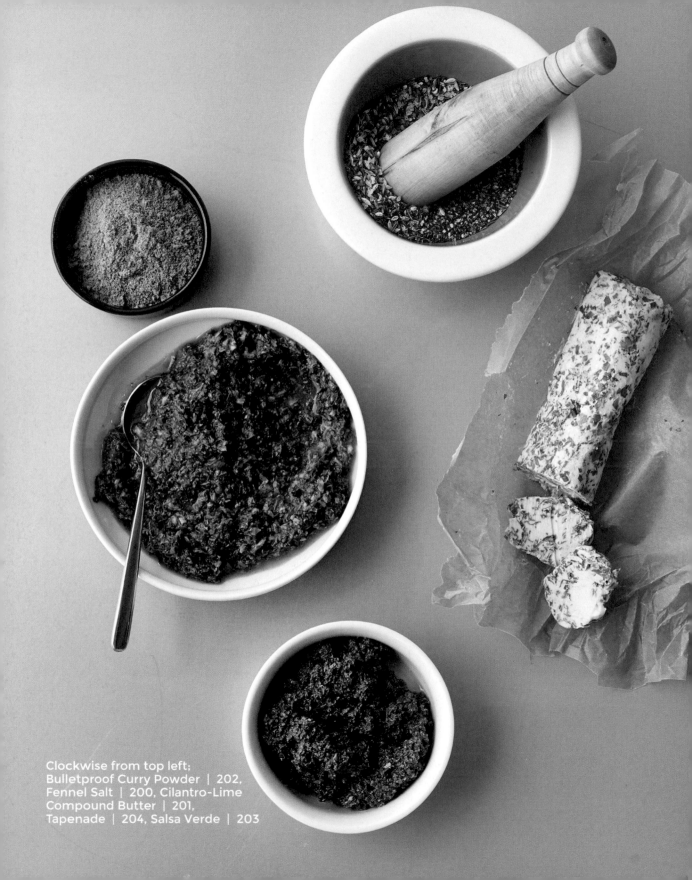

Clockwise from top left:
Bulletproof Curry Powder | 202,
Fennel Salt | 200, Cilantro-Lime
Compound Butter | 201,
Tapenade | 204, Salsa Verde | 203

UPGRADED BONE BROTH

This essential broth appeared in my first book, and it's so vital to being Bullet-proof that it needs to be here, too. Bone broth makes a great base for soup recipes, and hard-core fans even drink it straight for a high-performance shot of healthy animal fats!

3	medium carrots, cut into rough chunks
3	medium celery stalks, cut into rough chunks
2½	pounds assorted beef marrow bones from grass-fed beef
1	bouquet garni: your choice of fresh oregano, rosemary, thyme, sage, etc., tied in a bundle with kitchen twine
1 to 2	tablespoons apple cider vinegar
1	cup Bulletproof Upgraded Collagen Powder per 4 cups of broth (optional)
	Sea salt

In a large stockpot, lightly sauté the carrots and celery for a few minutes until translucent. Add the beef bones and bouquet garni and cover with water. Add the vinegar (it helps draw out the nutrients from the bones). Simmer over low heat (do not boil) for anywhere between 8 and 14 hours.

When your broth is a deep brown color and you are happy with the concentration of flavor, remove the bones and strain the vegetables out. If using collagen powder, add the amount appropriate to the amount of broth and stir until dissolved.

Add salt to taste, if desired, then store in canning jars in the refrigerator for future use.

ASIAN-STYLE BONE BROTH

MAKES ABOUT 8 CUPS

We serve this at the Bulletproof coffee shop in Santa Monica, and it's full of healthy animal proteins. It packs so much more collagen than any bone broth you could make, not including the Upgraded Collagen Powder.

1 tablespoon Bulletproof Brain Octane oil (or MCT or coconut oil)

3 medium carrots, cut into rough chunks

3 medium celery stalks, cut into rough chunks

1 bouquet garni: 2 scallions and 10 cilantro stems tied in a bundle with kitchen twine

2½ pounds assorted beef marrow bones from grass-fed beef

1 piece (2 inches) fresh ginger, peeled

1 large cinnamon stick (optional)

2 star anise (optional)

5 whole cloves (optional)

3 cardamom pods (optional)

¼ cup apple cider vinegar

1 cup Bulletproof Upgraded Collagen Powder per 4 cups of broth (optional)

Sea salt (optional)

In a large stockpot, heat the oil over medium-low heat. Add the carrots and celery and lightly sauté for a few minutes, until translucent.

Add the bouquet garni, beef bones, ginger, and (optional) spices and cover with cold water. Add the vinegar (this helps draw the nutrients from the bones). Bring to a boil, then immediately reduce the heat to low and simmer (do not boil) for 8 to 14 hours. Occasionally use a skimmer to skim off any particles or oil.

When your broth is a deep brown color and you are happy with the concentration of flavor, remove the bones and strain the vegetables out. If using collagen powder, add the amount appropriate to the amount of broth and stir until dissolved.

Add salt to taste, if desired, then store in canning jars, in the refrigerator for future use.

CARROT AND GINGER SMOOTHIE SOUP

SERVES 1 OR 2

When I grew up, I never liked soup because it was watery with a few sad vegetables floating around—blenders sucked in the 1970s. Now you can get great flavor and fats, all blended to creamy perfection. Taking the time to lightly cook the carrots in a ginger-infused broth makes this comforting combo easy to digest. Remember to skip the protein powder if you're fasting.

1	cup canned coconut milk, well shaken
1½	cups water
2	cups carrot slices (¼ inch thick)
1	tablespoon grated fresh ginger
½	teaspoon sea salt
2 to 4	tablespoons grass-fed unsalted butter (use hunger as your guide)
1 to 4	teaspoons apple cider vinegar (to taste)
2	tablespoons high-quality heat-stable protein powder (like Bulletproof Upgraded Collagen Powder)

In a medium saucepan, combine the coconut milk, water, carrots, ginger, and salt. Bring to a boil and immediately reduce to a simmer. Cook until the carrots start to soften, 5 to 7 minutes. Transfer carefully to a blender. Cover the blender lid with a cloth (in case the lid leaks) and blend until smooth. Add the butter and blend again. Add the vinegar and adjust the seasoning. Lastly add the protein powder and lightly blend until the protein is mixed in. Serve warm.

RICE SOUP WITH BOK CHOY AND CASHEWS

SERVES 2

For extra protein, this soup is great topped with shredded Duck Confit (page 98). When protein-fasting, omit the cashews.

2¾ to 3 cups Upgraded Bone Broth (page 147) or beef stock

¼ cup short-grain rice

1 teaspoon minced fresh ginger

¼ teaspoon ground turmeric

Sea salt

1 head bok choy, trimmed, sliced crosswise into ¼-inch-wide strips, leaves and stalks separated

1 tablespoon ground cashews or almonds, or almond meal (optional)

Cilantro leaves, for serving

Lime wedges, for serving

In a saucepot, combine the broth, rice, ginger, turmeric, and salt to taste. Bring to a simmer over medium heat. Reduce the heat to low, cover, and cook until the rice is tender, about 20 minutes. Uncover, add the bok choy stems, and cook, stirring, for 2 minutes. Add the bok choy greens and cook 1 minute more.

Serve the soup topped with ground cashews (if using), cilantro, and a squeeze of lime.

CAULIFLOWER AND CASHEW SOUP

SERVES 1 OR 2

Overlooked for years, cauliflower comes into its own with this flavorful soup with cashews. I came to appreciate cashews when I was a raw vegan because I was always starving for fat, and I could put them in desserts and use them to thicken things up. I think that they should be ahead of the more popular garbanzos in healthful cooking.

1 medium head cauliflower, cut into small florets

2 sprigs of rosemary

1/2 teaspoon sea salt

1/2 cup cashew nuts

1 teaspoon finely grated lemon zest

1/8 teaspoon cayenne pepper (optional)

2 tablespoons grass-fed unsalted butter

1 tablespoon fresh lemon juice

In a saucepan fitted with a steamer insert, bring 1 inch of water to a simmer over medium-high heat. Add the cauliflower and rosemary, cover, and steam until soft, 10 to 15 minutes. Discard the rosemary and let the cauliflower cool for a few moments. Scoop out 1/2 cup of the steamer water. Transfer the hot water and cauliflower to a blender. Add the salt, cashews, lemon zest, and cayenne (if using) and blend until smooth. Add the butter and blend again. Stir in the lemon juice. Adjust the seasoning to taste.

CHILLED AVOCADO AND CUCUMBER SOUP

I love this recipe because you can have it for lunch or dinner and it travels easily. Avocado is one of the best salad ingredients as a soup because it really holds up. It's a great make-ahead lunch, even for entertaining.

1	large cucumber, peeled and cut into chunks (about 2 cups)
1	large avocado, pitted, peeled, and cut into chunks
2	scallions, coarsely chopped
1	tablespoon fresh dill, plus sprigs for serving
1	teaspoon sea salt
1	teaspoon grated lemon zest
2	tablespoons fresh lemon juice
¼	cup water
1 or 2	tablespoons grass-fed full-fat yogurt (optional)

In a blender, combine all the ingredients except the yogurt and blend until smooth. Add more water if you want to make the soup thinner. Adjust the seasoning. This soup is great to serve immediately but even better if you chill for at least 2 hours and up to 6 hours. Garnish with dill sprigs and, if desired, top each serving with a tablespoon of yogurt.

COLD LETTUCE SOUP

SERVES 1 OR 2

I know it sounds crazy, but don't knock it 'til you try it. This is an opportunity to play around with various lettuce varietals; just be sure to buy organic. I always add Brain Octane oil to the blender to bring out flavor in this recipe. If you don't tolerate yogurt, play with increasing other fats.

4	cups loosely packed shredded assorted salad greens, such as romaine lettuce, arugula, escarole, lamb's lettuce (aka mâche), etc.
½	cup grass-fed full-fat yogurt
¼	cup fresh mint leaves
2	scallions, chopped (optional)
½	teaspoon sea salt
1 to 4	teaspoons apple cider vinegar (to taste)
2 to 4	tablespoons grass-fed unsalted butter (use your hunger as a guide)

In a blender, combine all the ingredients and blend until smooth and creamy. Add up to ¼ cup water to thin if desired. Serve chilled.

SIMPLE GREEN BULLETPROOF SOUP

SERVES 1 OR 2

There are endless varieties of simple green smoothies like this one. It's really the most versatile recipe ever. Warming the vegetables brings out more nutrients than blending veggies raw. Plus, you can add any meat you want to complete the flavor. I also like to substitute fennel for celery.

3	cups spinach
1	celery stalk
½	apple (optional)
1	cup coarsely chopped zucchini (1 medium)
1	cup water, freshly boiled
1 to 4	teaspoons apple cider vinegar (to taste)
2 to 4	teaspoons grass-fed unsalted butter (use your hunger as a guide)
1 to 2	tablespoons Bulletproof Brain Octane oil (or MCT or coconut oil)

In a high-speed blender, combine all the ingredients until smooth and creamy.

COCONUT-CRANBERRY SOUP

SERVES 1

This is delicious, but be sure you get dried cranberries that are sweetened naturally without corn syrup. You want to avoid hidden sugars at all cost. If you can find young Thai coconuts in a local market, by all means use them. Their fresh flavor is a treat.

1/3 cup dried cranberries

1 cup filtered water, freshly boiled

1 piece (1 inch) fresh ginger, peeled and thinly sliced

1 cup chopped peeled cucumber

2 teaspoons ground cinnamon

1 teaspoon fresh thyme leaves

1 can (14 ounces) coconut milk (or 1 young Thai coconut, meat and water)

1 tablespoon Bulletproof Brain Octane oil (or MCT or coconut oil)

1 tablespoon chopped almonds or pecans, for serving

1 teaspoon thinly sliced fresh mint, for serving

In a small saucepan, combine the dried cranberries and hot water and set aside to rehydrate for 10 minutes. Add the ginger, cucumber, cinnamon, and thyme. Bring to a boil, then immediately reduce to a simmer and cook over medium-low heat for 10 minutes. Transfer to a blender. Cover the blender lid with a cloth (in case the lid leaks) and blend until smooth. Add the coconut milk and Brain Octane oil and blend again until creamy. Serve with chopped nuts and mint.

BOK CHOY ANISE SOUP

SERVES 1 OR 2

I discovered this recipe because I would buy the vegetables in season at the farmers' market and sometimes I had more bok choy than I knew what to do with.

- 1 small napa cabbage, lower white portions only, thinly sliced
- 1 head bok choy, white stalks only, thinly sliced
- 4 scallions, white parts only, thinly sliced
- 2 cups water
- 1 teaspoon ground coriander
- $\frac{1}{4}$ teaspoon ground anise
- 1 teaspoon sea salt

  Juice of $\frac{1}{2}$ lemon
- 1 tablespoon expeller-pressed coconut oil
- 1 tablespoon coconut butter
- 1 tablespoon Bulletproof Brain Octane oil (or MCT or coconut oil)

In a medium saucepan, combine the cabbage, bok choy, and scallions and cook over low heat, stirring often, until fragrant, about 4 minutes. Add the water, coriander, anise, sea salt, and lemon juice. Cover and cook until the vegetables are just tender, about 10 minutes. Transfer to a blender. Cover the blender lid with a cloth (in case the lid leaks) and blend until smooth. Add the coconut oil, coconut butter, and Brain Octane oil and blend again until smooth and uniform.

BROCCOLI AND LEEK SOUP

SERVES 2, WITH LEFTOVERS

This tastes like a classic cream of broccoli soup so it's always satisfying and comforting. The leeks stand in for that stronger member of the allium family, garlic, so you get the flavor without the side effects.

1 tablespoon Bulletproof Brain Octane oil (or MCT or coconut oil)

1 leek, well washed and thinly sliced

1 celery stalk, thinly sliced

1 bunch broccoli, stems peeled and finely chopped, florets cut into $1/2$-inch pieces

2 cups water

1 teaspoon apple cider vinegar

2 teaspoons ground fenugreek

1 teaspoon coarse sea salt

$1/4$ cup coconut oil

$1/2$ cup ghee or grass-fed butter

In a medium saucepan, heat the Brain Octane oil over medium heat. Add the leek, celery, and broccoli stems and cook, stirring often, until softened, 3 to 4 minutes. Add the water, broccoli florets, vinegar, fenugreek, and salt. Cover and cook until the broccoli is tender, about 10 minutes. Transfer the broccoli mixture to a blender. Cover the blender lid with a cloth (in case the lid leaks) and blend until smooth. Add the coconut oil and ghee and puree again until smooth.

FENNEL EGG SOUP

SERVES 2

The eggs give this soup a Bulletproof blast of protein and texture.

1   leek, white and light green parts only, well washed and thinly sliced

1   small head cauliflower, cut into small florets

1   zucchini or yellow summer squash, thinly sliced

3   asparagus spears, trimmed and thinly sliced

1   small fennel bulb, trimmed and finely chopped

2   cups water

1   teaspoon apple cider vinegar

1   teaspoon sea salt

4   large pastured egg yolks

¼   cup ghee or grass-fed unsalted butter

1   tablespoon Bulletproof Brain Octane oil (or MCT or coconut oil)

In a medium pot, cook the leek over medium-low heat, stirring occasionally, until fragrant, about 3 minutes. Add the cauliflower, zucchini, asparagus, fennel, water, vinegar, and salt. Bring to a simmer, cover, and cook for 10 minutes, until the vegetables soften. Transfer to a blender. Cover the blender lid with a cloth (in case the lid leaks) and blend until smooth. Add the egg yolks, ghee, and Brain Octane oil and blend again until smooth and creamy.

FENNEL AND BROCCOLI SMOOTHIE SOUP WITH RICE

SERVES 1 OR 2

Fennel is an underused, underappreciated vegetable. Crunchy and slightly sweet, it's also a digestive aid. When I make this recipe, I love to put ground lamb on top of it.

2 tablespoons Bulletproof Brain Octane oil (or MCT or coconut oil)

1 cup fennel slices (¼ inch thick)

1 cup small broccoli florets

1 cup leek slices (¼ inch thick)

1 teaspoon fresh thyme leaves

¾ teaspoon sea salt

2 cups water

1 cup cooked white rice

2 tablespoons grass-fed unsalted butter

In a medium saucepan, heat the oil over medium-low heat. Add the fennel, broccoli, leeks, thyme, and salt and cook until the vegetables soften and go translucent. Add the water, cover, and simmer until vegetables are becoming tender, about 15 minutes. Stir in the cooked rice (or, if you prefer the rice whole, add it at the end, after the soup is blended). Transfer the mixture to a blender. Cover the blender lid with a cloth (in case the lid leaks) and blend until smooth. Add the butter and blend again. Adjust the seasoning before serving.

VIETNAMESE-STYLE FISH CHOWDER

SERVES 1 OR 2

This soup is typically served for breakfast in Vietnam, and the fragrant broth makes a perfect weekend brunch. When making my version of this dish, you'll want to avoid fish sauce, which is the highest histamine food you can buy.

1 can (14 ounces) coconut milk

1 teaspoon Bulletproof Curry Powder (page 202), optional

½ cup water

1 teaspoon grated fresh ginger

½ teaspoon sea salt

½ jalapeño pepper, seeded and finely chopped (optional)

¼ bunch cilantro, stems and leaves separated (roughly ¼ cup leaves)

1 wild haddock fillet (½ pound), or any sustainable wild-caught white fish

1 cup finely chopped boy choy

Juice of 1 lime

In a medium saucepan, whisk together the coconut milk and curry powder and stir in the water. Add the ginger, salt, jalapeño (if using), and cilantro stems. Bring to a boil, them immediately reduce to a simmer and cook for 15 minutes. With a slotted spoon, fish out the cilantro stems. Add the haddock and simmer until just cooked and starting to flake, about 5 minutes. Add the bok choy, stirring gently to break up the fish. Season with salt to taste. Stir in the lime juice and serve with cilantro leaves on top.

THAI FISH SOUP

SERVES 2

Turmeric gives this a wonderful color; fresh ginger and basil give it a Thai twist.

3 carrots, 1 finely chopped, 2 very thinly sliced

3 celery stalks, 1 finely chopped, 2 very thinly sliced

1 small head napa cabbage, thinly sliced

1 cup canned coconut milk, well shaken

1 piece (1 inch) fresh ginger, peeled and minced

2 teaspoons ground annatto (achiote) seeds

1 bay leaf

$\frac{1}{2}$ teaspoon ground turmeric

6 ounces Petrale sole fillet, cut into $\frac{3}{4}$-inch pieces

1 teaspoon coarse sea salt

$\frac{1}{4}$ cup coconut oil

1 tablespoon Bulletproof Brain Octane oil (or MCT or coconut oil)

1 tablespoon coconut butter

1 tablespoon almond butter

2 tablespoons chopped pitted black olives

Thinly sliced fresh basil, grated lime zest, and lime juice for serving

In a medium pot, cook the finely chopped carrots and finely chopped celery over medium heat until fragrant, about 3 minutes. Add the sliced carrots and celery, the cabbage, coconut milk, ginger, annatto seed, bay leaf, turmeric, sole, and salt. Cover and cook until the vegetables are tender and the fish is just cooked, about 10 minutes. Removing the bay leaf, transfer the soup (fish and all) to a blender. Cover the blender lid with a cloth (in case the lid leaks) and blend until smooth. Add the coconut oil, Brain Octane oil, coconut butter, almond butter, and olives, and puree until emulsified. Serve garnished with basil, lime zest, and lime juice.

FENNEL LEMONGRASS SOUP WITH SALMON

SERVES 2

After 10 years of making these soups, I've never grown tired of them. Using a vegetable with flavor like fennel you can do almost anything. Here I use fennel and lemongrass. For this recipe, use homemade broth (not just chicken stock). You can add Bulletproof Upgraded Collagen Powder if you want more protein. The creamy flavor of the fennel base stands up well to salmon, but you can substitute any Bulletproof fish, such as hake or tilapia, if you prefer.

2 teaspoons Bulletproof Brain Octane oil (or MCT or coconut oil)

1 leek, well washed, white and light green parts only, coarsely chopped (optional)

1 piece (1½ inches) fresh ginger, peeled and sliced

1 stalk lemongrass, trimmed of root and tops, cut into 3 pieces

1 kaffir lime leaf, stemmed, or 1 tablespoon grated lime zest

1 teaspoon ground turmeric

3 cups chicken stock or Upgraded Bone Broth (page 147)

1½ cups canned coconut milk, well shaken

2 fennel bulbs, trimmed, cored, and cut crosswise into ½-inch-thick pieces

Sea salt

1 pound salmon, skin removed and cut into 1-inch cubes

2 ounces spinach leaves

In a medium pot, combine the oil, leek (if using), and ginger. Cook gently over medium heat, stirring often, for 2 minutes. Add the lemongrass, lime leaf, turmeric, stock, and coconut milk. Bring to a simmer and cook for about 10 minutes to infuse with the aromatics. Add the fennel and cook, uncovered, until tender, about 6 minutes.

Remove the lemongrass and lime leaf. Transfer the soup to a blender. Cover the blender lid with a cloth (in case the lid leaks) and blend until smooth. Season with salt to taste. Return the soup to the pot and bring to a simmer. Add the salmon and cook, uncovered, until the salmon is just cooked, about 2 minutes. Remove the pan from heat and stir in the spinach. Season with salt to taste.

CHAPTER 8

LATTES AND SMOOTHIES

I think this is one of the most exciting recipe chapters in the book. More than in any other chapter, I broke out of the expected parameters for what a recipe should be. Mainly because I introduce a number of warm smoothies, which, sure, if you want to be technical, can (and should) be considered soups as well. I eat the flavors I like when I like them and don't worry about whether something fits traditional notions of when it should be enjoyed based on temperature, or sweet versus savory.

The recipes in this chapter start with my original hot drink: Bulletproof Coffee, followed by my take on a very popular latte. Many of us have outgrown "regular" coffee. Thanks to a certain coffee chain, many have become accustomed to flavored, infused coffee drinks and, in particular, a pumpkin something that sweeps the nation every autumn. The good news is that I've created my own Bulletproof riff on that popular concoction, but with all the benefits your body demands. You might not expect that using butternut squash could deliver the same amazing, autumnal flavor, but wait until you try it. With my Upgraded Coffee beans, rich butter, the harvest flavor of squash, a little aromatic cinnamon, and some stevia for sweetness, it's everything you love about fall without sacrificing your commitment to become Bulletproof. Remember, you really don't have to give up anything you love. With a little creativity, you can enjoy all your favorite seasonal treats.

Next up are some less-caffeinated but still powerful drinks: my upgraded hot chocolate and green tea latte.

A couple of overall tips from my first book for the coffee-based recipes: An immersion blender works fine if you don't have a high-powered blender handy, but if you are using a blender, pour hot tap water into it to preheat it while the coffee brews. Empty the hot water when the coffee is ready, then add all the ingredients. And you can brew the coffee whichever way you prefer, but I recommend using a metal-mesh filter if you're using a drip coffeemaker, or a French press.

It's surprising that more people don't enjoy warm smoothies; drinking something cold in the morning is jarring at best, and outright awful if you're in the middle of a harsh winter. It's also a shock to the system, yet somehow it's just what we do—blend up a bunch of fruit at temperatures so icy we can't even taste it and we get brain freeze. Suffice to say: I think you're going to love the warm smoothies in this section.

There are some cold smoothies here, too, and they certainly have their time and place, but the warm ones work year-round. They're a convenient, easy vehicle for a big dose of nutrients and fat. Besides that, there are some supernutritious foods that work well in a smoothie, but really shouldn't be eaten raw—like kale. Most people would throw kale into a cold smoothie with fruit and other greens, but if you know your Bulletproof rules, you already know you want to cook out the oxalic acid, a naturally occurring toxin that exists to fend off predators in the natural world. I also cook the carrots in my Carrot and Ginger Smoothie Soup, on page 149 in Chapter 7 (which could really go in this chapter, too!), to soften up the texture and make it easier to digest. If you think about it, it's not really possible to properly blend a carrot; it just doesn't get supersmooth unless it's juiced. By cooking it first, you'll achieve a supersmooth, creamy result, and when it's warm, it's over-the-top tasty. As with everything Bulletproof, you don't need to cook it much—just a light simmer or a steam is all it takes. No roasting necessary.

As far as adding protein to smoothies, I tend to favor whey or collagen. This is partially because some people are nervous about using raw eggs, but more so because protein powder is just so easy. We live in busy times, and protein powder packs a massive nutritional punch. It has no discernible taste, it's easy to store, and it won't go bad quickly. What's not to love? For our modern lifestyle, it's a superfood we should embrace.

For fats, of course I also use my tried-and-true favorite sources: MCT oil, coconut oil, and grass-fed butter. They're all great options, though butter makes everything taste so good and rich, it tends to be a favor-ite. I love it in the Warm Sweet Potato and Citrus Smoothie (page 170), which is really a food fit for the gods. It sounds like an odd combination at first, but trust me, this is a combination that will blow you away. I use up to 4 tablespoons of butter in mine, but if you're new to eating Bulletproof, you can start with 2 and let your hunger and cravings dictate how and when you add more. Butter is rich, and if you dive right in it could throw your system for a loop. The great thing is, the butter is so filling and so comforting, it's a warm meal to start your day—even if it's in the form of a smoothie!—and it will keep you energized all day long.

The last thing I'll say about warm smoothies is that the cooking process allows a nice infusion of flavors. Say you're working with coconut and cinnamon; the heating process lets the ingredients take on more flavor so your smoothie is that much tastier.

And now, the recipe that began it all and begins every day: Bulletproof Coffee.

BULLETPROOF COFFEE

SERVES 1

This is my centerpiece recipe. It's how you start your day and where the Bulletproof diet was born. Incorporate the grass-fed butter and Brain Octane oil gradually into your morning Bulletproof upgraded coffee. Start with 1 tablespoon of butter, working up to 2 tablespoons over the course of several days. For the oil, work up to 1 to 2 tablespoons over several days.

2½	heaping tablespoons freshly ground Bulletproof Upgraded Coffee beans or your best alternative—the cleanest beans you can find: Arabica, single-origin, high-grown (high-altitude), washed (or wet) process beans
1	cup filtered water, freshly boiled
1	teaspoon Bulletproof Brain Octane oil (or MCT or coconut oil)
1 to 2	tablespoons grass-fed unsalted butter

Brew the coffee with the water according to your preferred brewing method. Transfer the coffee to the blender along with the Brain Octane oil and butter and puree until smooth, emulsified, and frothy, about 20 seconds.

BULLETPROOF BUTTERNUT LATTE

SERVES 1 OR 2

Give your morning coffee a powerful blast of beta-carotene with the warming winter addition of butternut squash. Please note: This recipe is not appropriate when you're doing Bulletproof Intermittent Fasting because it includes carbs.

2 cups piping-hot brewed Bulletproof Upgraded Coffee beans

Up to 2 tablespoons grass-fed unsalted butter (use your hunger as a guide)

Up to 2 tablespoons Bulletproof Brain Octane oil (or MCT or coconut oil) (use your hunger as a guide)

1 cup cooked butternut squash cubes

½ teaspoon ground cinnamon (optional)

Stevia or hardwood xylitol (optional)

In a blender, combine the coffee, butter, Brain Octane oil, and butternut squash. Cover the blender lid with a cloth (in case the lid leaks) and blend until there's a thick layer of foam on top, like a latte. If desired, add the cinnamon and sweetener to taste.

BULLETPROOF COCONUT HOT CHOCOLATE

SERVES 1 OR 2

The interesting ingredients here are cacao butter and vanilla powder. (Of course, I like using my Bulletproof Cacao Butter and Bulletproof VanillaMax.) It smells super chocolatey and it gives you a great boost from all those good fats and quality sourced ingredients. This is a decadent, pleasurable drink that kids can enjoy too.

2 cups canned coconut milk, well shaken

1 tablespoon cacao butter

3 tablespoons Bulletproof Chocolate Powder

1 teaspoon lab-tested, mold-free vanilla powder, such as Bulletproof VanillaMax

Liquid stevia

In a small saucepan, bring the coconut milk to a boil over medium high heat and immediately remove from the heat. Transfer to a blender and add the cacao butter, chocolate powder, and vanilla powder. Cover the blender lid with a cloth (in case the lid leaks) and blend until you have a creamy consistency with a layer of foam on top. Sweeten with stevia to taste.

GREEN TEA LATTE

This green tea latte is a mellow alternative to coffee and chocolate milk, both of which are heavier and bolder in flavor. Matcha tea and coconut milk are mild, and green tea has the incredible side benefit of supporting focus and concentration—it's been favored for centuries by Zen monks for meditation. On protein-fasting days, feel free to leave out the protein powder. I favor Bulletproof VanillaMax and Bulletproof Whey Protein powder; if you use other types, be sure the protein powder is heat stable.

1   cup canned coconut milk, well shaken

½   cup filtered water, freshly boiled

1   teaspoon pure matcha green tea powder

1   teaspoon lab-tested, mold-free vanilla powder, such as Bulletproof VanillaMax

2   tablespoons Bulletproof Upgraded Collagen Protein Powder (optional)

Stevia or hardwood xylitol (optional)

In a small saucepan, bring the coconut milk to a boil over medium-high heat and immediately remove from the heat. In a small cup, mix the hot water and matcha tea powder together. In a blender, combine the tea, coconut milk, and vanilla powder. Cover the blender lid with a cloth (in case the lid leaks) and blend until you have a creamy consistency with a layer of foam on top. If desired, for extra protein, add the protein powder and lightly blend until the protein is mixed in. Sweeten to taste.

WARM SWEET POTATO AND CITRUS SMOOTHIE

SERVES 1 OR 2

This is not an obvious combination, but it's a great breakfast that will keep you full for awhile. It's a rich, sweet, and slightly sour treat for protein-fasting days.

1	cup chopped cooked sweet potato
½	cup filtered water, freshly boiled
2	tangerines, peeled, seeded, and chopped
½	teaspoon sea salt
1 to 4	teaspoons apple cider vinegar (to taste)
2 to 4	tablespoons grass-fed unsalted butter (use hunger as your guide)
1 to 2	tablespoons Bulletproof Brain Octane oil (or MCT or coconut oil) (use hunger as your guide)

In a blender, combine all the ingredients and blend until creamy.

WARM STEAMED KALE AND PINEAPPLE SMOOTHIE

SERVES 1 OR 2

This recipe includes some sugar from the pineapple, but it's such a great way to get kale—it's so delicious. Please note: This is not a good choice for a ketosis day. Be sure to Bulletproof the warm smoothie by steaming and draining the kale to keep its oxalates low.

- 1 cup packed chopped kale leaves (center ribs removed)
- 1 cup chopped pineapple
- ½ avocado, peeled
- 1 teaspoon fresh lime juice
- 2 tablespoons high-quality heat-stable protein powder (optional)

In a saucepan fitted with a steamer insert, bring a cup or so of water to a simmer. Add the kale, cover, and steam until cooked, about 5 minutes. Transfer the kale to a blender. Measure out ¼ cup of the steaming water and add to the blender along with the pineapple, avocado, and lime juice and blend until smooth and creamy. Add more hot water if you want a thinner consistency. If desired, for extra protein, add the protein powder and lightly blend until the protein is mixed in.

COCONUT SMOOTHIE

SERVES 1 OR 2

What better way to incorporate coconut oil into your diet than this pure white smoothie?

1/2	cup unsweetened coconut flakes
2	cups canned coconut milk, well shaken
1 to 2	tablespoons Bulletproof Brain Octane oil (or MCT or coconut oil) (use your hunger as a guide)
1	teaspoon lab-tested, mold-free vanilla powder, such as Bulletproof VanillaMax
2	tablespoons Bulletproof Upgraded Collagen Protein Powder (optional)
	Stevia or hardwood xylitol

Preheat the oven to 300°F.

Spread the coconut in a baking pan and bake the coconut, stirring and watching carefully, until toasted (don't let it darken), about 3 minutes. Set aside a handful of flakes for garnish and transfer the rest to a blender.

To a blender, add the coconut milk, coconut oil, and vanilla powder and blend until the coconut breaks down and you have a creamy consistency, at least 1 minute. If desired, for extra protein, add the protein powder and lightly blend until the protein is mixed in. Sweeten to taste. Top with the reserved toasted coconut.

STRABERRIES AND CREAM SMOOTHIE

SERVES 2

Everyone needs a treat now and then, and it doesn't get much better than pure strawberries and cream.

2 cups strawberries (preferably in season from the farmers' market)

½ cup grass-fed cream (or coconut cream, if preferred)

1 teaspoon chopped fresh mint, plus sprigs for garnish

Stevia or hardwood xylitol (optional)

In a blender, combine the strawberries and cream and blend until smooth. Add the mint and blend again briefly. Add some water, if needed, to thin consistency. If desired, sweeten to taste. Garnish with a sprig of mint.

CHAPTER 9

DESSERTS

And here we are at desserts. Like the chapter on lattes and smoothies, I really love what's possible here because you'd think you have to make sacrifices when it comes to delicious, delectable treats. But if you know how to bring out the natural sweetness and smooth textures of Bulletproof foods, you can make desserts that I daresay taste even better than those laden with sugar and other antinutrient foods.

To state the obvious, there's no white sugar here—there's also no coconut sugar and no agave. But that doesn't mean there's no sweetness. If you're building a Bulletproof pantry, you can include xylitol, erythritol, and stevia to make pretty much anything you like. I find that xylitol and erythritol have pretty pronounced flavor profiles on their own (the former is tinny, the latter like burnt wood), but blending a mix of the two is a perfect solution for a broader flavor profile. I also use a little stevia here and there, but my half-and-half blend is my go-to solution for sweetener. In some cases, I also powdered the mixture in the blender, because they come in a coarse grain like a raw sugar. This is a good hack if you're trying to Bulletproof other recipes: You can powder xylitol and erythritol and they will work the same way as a product with a finer consistency. When you're sourcing xylitol, find the non-GMO variety and please note that it is extremely toxic to dogs. It can kill them. This has been the sad case in many homes where gum is left lying around, so please keep your xylitol (in whatever form) stored safely—for you, and your pets.

In addition to subbing in sweeteners for sugar, I find you can use the natural textures of many Bulletproof foods to enhance creaminess. Strawberries make a nice creamy sorbet, and when berries are tart (like raspberries), you can add beets for a super-sweet flavor and a luscious creamy texture. You can also use avocado to create rich, creamy texture and mouthfeel. The Vegan Chocolate Mousse (page 190) is a perfect example of just how velvety a Bulletproof dessert can be. Trust me, you're not going to feel you're missing out on anything.

I do use a little maple syrup, because I allow myself some moderation foods here and there, especially around the holidays if there's a certain flavor profile I'm trying to hit. "Very Dark" maple syrup is pure and it tastes amazing, so you need less of it and still get all the flavor you crave.

Another hack to remember when thinking about sweetening up desserts is that vanilla goes a long way in terms of replacing sweetness thanks to its aromatic quality. It satisfies, and provides that warm, fragrant suggestion of baked goods.

Honey is an interesting option for desserts because it's helpful for hacking sleep patterns. Now if you cook it, you denature it, so I just drizzle it—on fruits, crepes, whatever. Always look for honey that's raw, and try to support your local beekeeper (and your local bees), because that product will have beneficial properties and help treat allergies to your local environment. Since you're having dessert at the end of the day, this is perfect time to hack your sleep with a little added honey before bed.

If you're using fruit in your desserts, stick with what's seasonal. For example, if a recipe calls for strawberries but they're out of season, swap them out for an in-season berry. That way you're not only getting the ripest, freshest, best tasting berries, you're also reducing the likelihood of ingesting mold toxins that build up during food storage.

BULLETPROOF CUPCAKES

MAKES 20 CUPCAKES

I developed this recipe over a period of about 2 years and largely for my kids. My daughter, Anna, who's eight, still loves baking and I like to think it's because, before she was old enough to walk, she used to make these with me. Most Paleo-style desserts are simply too carby, but these can work with almost no carbs at all if you omit the rice flour. They taste amazing, and they're not dry or tough. The trick is to use whipped egg whites.

If you use erythritol, watch for its endothermic (strongly cooling) reaction with the proteins in the egg, which drops the temperature of the mixing bowl by about 20 degrees! If sweet rice flour is not available, just omit it; don't substitute regular rice flour, which will make the cupcakes taste gritty.

- **6** tablespoons erythritol
- **6** tablespoons xylitol
- **12** ounces dark chocolate (at least 85% cacao), chips or finely chopped bar
- **1½** sticks (6 ounces) grass-fed unsalted butter, at room temperature

  Pinch of pink Himalayan salt
- **6** large pastured eggs, at room temperature, separated
- **2** teaspoons lab-tested, mold-free vanilla powder, such as Bulletproof VanillaMax
- **1** teaspoon cocoa powder, such as Bulletproof Upgraded Chocolate Powder
- **1** tablespoon sweet rice flour

Position racks in the upper and lower thirds of the oven and preheat to 350°F. Line 20 cups of 2 muffin tins with paper liners.

Pulse the erythritol and xylitol in a blender until finely ground. Set aside.

In a small saucepan, bring about 2 cups water to a simmer over medium-low heat. Place the chocolate and butter in a large heatproof bowl that can sit on top of the saucepan but not directly touching the water. Place the bowl on the pan and stir occasionally until the chocolate and butter are completely melted, about 10 minutes. Remove from the heat and set aside to cool slightly.

In a stand mixer with the paddle attachment, beat together 6 tablespoons of the powdered erythritol/xylitol, the salt, and egg yolks on medium-high speed until the mixture is thick and pale, about 3 minutes. Using a rubber spatula, gently fold the yolk mixture into the melted chocolate and stir in the vanilla powder, cocoa powder, and sweet rice flour.

In a separate bowl, with an electric mixer, beat the egg whites on medium speed until soft peaks form. Slowly beat in the erythritol/xylitol, then increase the speed to medium-high and beat until medium peaks form.

Gently fold the egg white mixture into the chocolate mixture, one-third at a time, until combined. Using a ¼-cup ice cream scoop or cup measure, spoon the batter into the muffin cups. Bake until a toothpick inserted in the center of a cupcake comes out with a few moist crumbs, about 25 minutes. Let cool in the pan about 5 minutes before transferring to a cooling rack to cool completely.

BULLETPROOF "GET SOME" VANILLA ICE CREAM

SERVES 2

No Bulletproof book would be complete without a reference to this ice cream. I created this to restore my wife's fertility. An hour after you've eaten this food, you have everything necessary to make a baby. The only way to know if it works for you is to break out the ice cream maker (I like the Cuisinart one that uses a frozen bowl). The trick is the 10 drops of apple cider vinegar or lime juice. Please note: It's important that you use Bulletproof Brain Octane or MCT oil, not just coconut oil, because it changes the characteristics of the texture. If you're looking for extra protein, try some Bulletproof Upgraded Whey—just a couple tablespoons will make it a lighter texture.

4	large pastured eggs
4	large pastured egg yolks
1	teaspoon lab-tested, mold-free vanilla powder, such as Bulletproof VanillaMax
10	drops apple cider vinegar
7	tablespoons grass-fed unsalted butter
7	tablespoons coconut oil
3	tablespoons plus 2 teaspoons Bulletproof Brain Octane oil (or MCT or coconut oil)
5½	tablespoons xylitol or erythritol
	Up to ½ cup of water or ice (as needed)

In a blender, combine all the ingredients except the water/ice in a blender and blend until creamy. Add water or ice slowly and blend again—for a creamy consistency add water only until the mixture is the thickness of heavy cream. For an icier texture, add more water.

Pour the mixture into an ice cream maker and process according to the manufacturer's instructions. Transfer to a quart container and place in the freezer until frozen, about 2 hours or overnight.

BERRIES AND COCONUT CREAM

SERVES 2

One combination that almost anyone enjoys is heavy whipped cream and berries, but when you realize coconut cream has a different and preferable effect, it's easy to switch over. If you can't find coconut cream, you can strain out the watery part from a can of coconut milk and use what remains. You can also use a dash of xylitol, but just make sure it's dissolved into the watery part of the coconut milk before you drain it off or it will be gritty.

10	ounces mixed berries (such as blackberries, blueberries, and raspberries)
½	cup well chilled coconut cream
¼	teaspoon lab-tested, mold-free vanilla powder, such as Bulletproof VanillaMax
½ to 1	teaspoon fresh lemon juice
1 to 2	teaspoons maple syrup (optional)

Divide the berries between 2 bowls.

In a separate large bowl, combine the coconut milk, vanilla powder, lemon juice, and maple syrup (if using) and whisk to soft peaks.

Place dollops of the whipped coconut cream on top of the berries.

BULLETPROOF FRUIT SALAD

SERVES 1 OR 2

This is creamier than a normal fruit salad because of the avocado. Paired with vitamin C-rich citrus, avocados up the Bulletproof factor of this dessert. Please note, the dark green part just inside the skin is highest in antioxidants, so scrape inside the peel for all the goodness.

1¼	cups pineapple cubes (8 ounces)
1	orange, segmented (see How to Segment Citrus, page 85), juice reserved
1	teaspoon fresh lime juice
1	teaspoon raw honey
½	avocado, peeled and cubed
1	tablespoon thinly sliced fresh mint
1	tablespoon unsweetened coconut flakes

In a small bowl, combine the pineapple, orange segments and juice, lime juice, honey, avocado, and mint. Gently stir to combine. Top with the coconut.

RASPBERRY-BEET SORBET

SERVES 2

This is a great option for dessert when you are adding carbohydrates, as the beets are a good choice for an end-of-day carb. They also make this sorbet extra creamy—and the color is amazing! Please note, too many beets will increase oxalic acid levels, but a little bit increases an otherwise healthy state.

$\frac{1}{2}$	pound beets
$\frac{1}{4}$	cup erythritol
$\frac{1}{4}$	cup xylitol
12	ounces raspberries (about 3 cups)
2	tablespoons Bulletproof Brain Octane oil (or MCT or coconut oil)
$1\frac{1}{2}$	teaspoons vanilla powder
1	tablespoon fresh lemon juice
	Pinch of sea salt

Preheat the oven to 325°F.

Place the beets in an 8 x 8-inch baking dish with ¼ cup water. Cover and bake until tender when pierced with a knife, about 1 hour. Allow to cool, then slip off the peels.

In a blender, process the erythritol and xylitol until powdered. Add the beets, raspberries, oil, vanilla powder, lemon juice, and salt. Process until smooth. Push mixture through a fine-mesh sieve set over a medium bowl to get rid of the seeds (discard them).

Chill the mixture for 1 hour, then process in an ice cream maker according to the manufacturer's instructions. Chill sorbet in freezer for 1 hour before serving.

STRAWBERRY SEMIFREDDO

SERVES 2, WITH LEFTOVERS

This is basically a light custard. It takes a little work, but it's delicious and you'll definitely impress your guests. Make sure your strawberries are organic and local if you can find them since strawberries are often heavily sprayed with pesticides. If you're like me, you might skip the seeding step, but technically that leads to a smoother result.

1	can (14 ounces) coconut milk, well shaken
¼	cup erythritol
¼	cup xylitol
2	pounds strawberries
1	tablespoon Bulletproof Brain Octane oil (or MCT or coconut oil)
	Grated zest of 2 limes
3	large pastured egg yolks
	Pinch of sea salt
½	teaspoon lab-tested, mold-free vanilla powder, such as Bulletproof VanillaMax

Place the coconut milk in the freezer for 15 minutes, until cold.

Set up a cold-water bath: Fill a large bowl halfway with ice water. Line a 9 x 5-inch loaf pan with plastic wrap with a 2-inch overhang on each side.

Pulse the erythritol and xylitol in a blender until finely ground. Set aside.

In a blender, combine 1½ pounds of the strawberries, the oil, lime zest, and ¼ cup of the powdered erythritol/xylitol and puree until smooth. Push the mixture through a fine-mesh strainer set over a medium bowl to get rid of the seeds (discard them). Measure out ½ cup of the puree and refrigerate until serving.

Fill a medium saucepan with 1 inch of water and bring to a simmer over medium heat. In a large heatproof bowl that will fit over the saucepan, beat together the egg yolks, remaining ¼ cup powdered erythritol/xylitol, and salt. Place the bowl over, but not touching, the simmering water and whisk constantly until the mixture starts to thicken and form thick ribbons, about 6 minutes. Transfer the bowl immediately to the cold-water bath. Allow to cool briefly.

Meanwhile, in a bowl, with an electric mixer, beat the chilled coconut milk and vanilla powder on medium-high speed to soft peaks, about 5 minutes.

Fold 2 cups of the whipped coconut cream into the cooled egg mixture, then fold in the strawberry puree from the medium bowl until swirls form. Pour the semifreddo base into the prepared loaf pan, tapping the pan to remove bubbles. Fold the plastic over the cream and freeze for 6 hours or overnight.

Remove the pan from the freezer and allow to soften slightly, about 45 minutes.

Meanwhile, quarter the remaining strawberries and set aside.

Cut the semifreddo into 1-inch-thick slices with a serrated knife. Serve with the reserved ½ cup strawberry puree, quartered berries, and a spoonful of remaining coconut cream.

RASPBERRY CLAFOUTIS

SERVES 4

One of the food consultants on this book gave me the fancy French name for this dessert. Personally, I'm still working on pronouncing it right. It's *cla-foo-tee*. Please note: You can substitute blackberries for the raspberries, and you can use as much as 16 ounces of these micronutrient-dense, antioxidant-rich berries in this delicious creation. Just be sure to use very high-quality berries to avoid mold toxin.

1	teaspoon grass-fed unsalted butter, for buttering the dish
12 to 16	ounces raspberries
3	large pastured eggs
1¼	cups canned coconut milk, well shaken
½	cup sweet rice flour
¼	teaspoon vanilla powder
	Grated zest of 1 lemon
¼	cup erythritol
¼	cup xylitol
	Pinch of sea salt

Preheat the oven to 350°F. Butter a shallow 2-quart baking pan, pie pan, or tart pan.

Place the berries on the bottom of the buttered pan.

In a large bowl, whisk together the eggs, coconut milk, rice flour, vanilla powder, lemon zest, erythritol, xylitol, and salt until smooth.

Pour the batter over the raspberries and bake until puffed slightly and set, 35 to 40 minutes. Let the clafoutis cool briefly for about 10 minutes before serving.

PINEAPPLE GRANITA

SERVES 2

Packed with vitamin C and garnished with antioxidant-rich raspberries, this dessert is a light and refreshing choice for carb days. You'll be amazed what the vanilla does for this dish. It really makes the flavor pop. I've also been known to dab a little Brain Octane oil in the blending phase to activate the fat receptors in my taste buds.

- 1 small pineapple, peeled and cored
- 1 tablespoon fresh lime juice
- 1 tablespoon raw honey or xylitol
- $\frac{1}{8}$ teaspoon lab-tested, mold-free vanilla powder, such as Bulletproof VanillaMax
- 2 teaspoons finely chopped fresh mint, for garnish

  Raspberries, for garnish

In a blender, combine the pineapple, lime juice, honey, and vanilla powder and let stand for 5 minutes to draw out juices. Then pulse to a thick but textured puree. Transfer to an 8 x 8-inch 2-quart freezerproof container. Place in the freezer and freeze, stirring every 30 minutes, until slushy and almost firm, about 3 hours.

Scrape the granita with a fork and divide it between 2 bowls. Serve garnished with mint and raspberries.

CHOCOLATE-COCONUT TRUFFLES

MAKES 6 TRUFFLES

You can substitute walnuts or any other nut for a twist, or roll the finished balls in unsweetened coconut flakes for a more intense coconut flavor. These bites are superfilling and they keep really well. Just know that, inevitably, something will end up on your face.

1/4	cup coconut cream (from the top of an unshaken 14-ounce can of coconut milk)
1	tablespoon raw cacao powder, such as Bulletproof Upgraded Chocolate Powder
2	ounces dark chocolate (at least 85% cacao), chopped
1/4	teaspoon lab-tested, mold-free vanilla powder, such as Bulletproof VanillaMax
1	tablespoon cold water
1	tablespoon grass-fed unsalted butter
1 1/2	teaspoons raw honey or xylitol
3	tablespoons finely ground raw almonds
	Sea salt

In a saucepan, bring 1 cup water to a simmer over medium heat. In a heatproof medium bowl that will fit over the saucepan without touching the water, combine the coconut cream, cacao powder, chocolate, vanilla powder, and 1 tablespoon cold water. Place the bowl over the simmering water and stir occasionally until the chocolate is melted, about 4 minutes. Remove the bowl from the pan and let the chocolate mixture cool slightly (to body temperature), about 10 minutes.

Whisk the butter and honey into the melted chocolate until combined. Stir in 2 tablespoons of the almonds. Refrigerate to chill, about 1 hour.

Form the mixture into six 1½-inch balls and roll in the remaining 1 tablespoon ground almonds. Top with a sprinkling of salt.

CHOCOLATE-DIPPED PEARS

SERVES 2

Pears are a high-fructose fruit so enjoy this dish when you're not having other fructose during the day. I've also done this with strawberries and it's wonderful. These are not to be eaten often but should be enjoyed fully when you do.

2 ounces dark chocolate (at least 85% cacao), coarsely chopped

1 tablespoon grass-fed unsalted butter, at room temperature

2 ripe but firm Bosc or Anjou pears, well washed and dried

Topping: 1 tablespoon ground nuts (almonds, walnuts, or hazelnuts), cocoa nibs, or unsweetened coconut flakes

Coarse sea salt

Line a plate or small baking sheet with parchment paper and set aside.

Bring 1 inch of water to a simmer in a small pot. In a small heatproof bowl that sits over the pot without touching the water, melt the chocolate, stirring occasionally until three-fourths melted, 8 to 10 minutes. Remove the bowl from the pan and stir the chocolate until it is fully melted. Stir in the butter until well combined. The chocolate should be melted but not hot.

Tilt the bowl slightly to make a deeper pool of chocolate. Dip each pear bottom into the chocolate. Sprinkle the chocolate with the topping of choice and coarse salt and place on the parchment. Chill in refrigerator until the chocolate is set, about 20 minutes.

VEGAN CHOCOLATE MOUSSE

SERVES 2

You didn't think you'd find vegan recipes in this book, did you? It's possible to have high-fat vegan food, especially when you use avocado instead of eggs. This recipe is amazing, plain and simple. It makes the perfect finish for an omega-3-rich dinner like the Fennel Lemongrass Soup with Salmon (page 162).

6	tablespoons coconut cream (from the top of an unshaken 14-ounce can of coconut milk)
4	tablespoons coconut liquid (from the bottom of the can of coconut milk)
1/2	teaspoon lab-tested, mold-free vanilla powder, such as Bulletproof VanillaMax
2	tablespoons stevia
4	ounces dark chocolate (at least 85% cacao), broken into 1-inch pieces
1/4	teaspoon coarse sea salt
1	Hass avocado, pitted and peeled

In a double boiler or in a heatproof bowl set over a saucepan of barely simmering water (medium-low heat), combine the coconut cream, coconut liquid, vanilla powder, stevia, chocolate, and salt, stirring gently until melted, 8 to 10 minutes. Transfer to a blender, add the avocado, and puree until smooth. Serve at room temperature or chill slightly for 15 minutes.

COCONUT CREPES WITH CITRUS SALAD

SERVES 2

Crepes are hard to do without carbs because they taste like fried eggs. These use sweet rice flour to hold them together and taste like real crepes. This is amazing as a dessert. You can also serve them with chocolate, of course. The recipe makes six crepes, so it's perfect for sharing on date night. And a little practice flipping them beforehand makes the presentation all the more impressive.

4 tablespoons grass-fed unsalted butter or ghee, gently melted

½ cup sweet rice flour (spooned and leveled)

2 large pastured eggs, at room temperature

¼ cup canned coconut milk, well shaken

2 tablespoons water

Pinch of sea salt

2 oranges, segmented (see How to Segment Citrus, page 85)

1 teaspoon raw honey, for drizzling (optional)

In a blender, combine 3 tablespoons of the melted butter, the rice flour, eggs, coconut milk, water, and salt. Blend until frothy and well blended, about 1 minute. Chill the batter for 1 hour.

Heat a 9-inch nonstick skillet or crepe pan over medium-low heat with just enough of the remaining melted butter to lightly coat. Pour ¼ cup batter into pan, swirling the pan to distribute the batter evenly. Cook undisturbed for 2 minutes, then carefully flip the crepe and cook on the second side for 1 minute more. Repeat to make 5 more crepes, adding butter to the pan as needed.

Serve the crepes with orange segments and, if desired, a drizzle of honey.

PUMPKIN FLAN

SERVES 8

Enjoy this dessert at the holidays when you are in maintenance mode. Real maple syrup is a fine low-fructose sweetener, so long as it is enjoyed only on special occasions and not daily. Be sure to purchase canned unsweetened pumpkin puree, not pumpkin pie filling, which is full of added sugar!

Bulletproof Brain Octane oil (or MCT or coconut oil) oil, for greasing the ramekins

3 cups coconut milk, well shaken

3 large pastured eggs

2 large pastured egg yolks

1 teaspoon ground cinnamon

$3/4$ teaspoon ground ginger

$1/2$ teaspoon coarse sea salt

$1/2$ teaspoon lab-tested, mold-free vanilla powder, such as Bulletproof VanillaMax

1 cup canned unsweetened pumpkin puree

$1/3$ cup high-quality "Very Dark" maple syrup, plus 2 tablespoons for serving

$1/4$ cup xylitol

Preheat the oven to 350°F. Grease the insides of eight 6-ounce ramekins with Brain Octane oil. Place the ramekins in a roasting pan large enough to hold them without touching.

In a blender, combine the coconut milk, whole eggs, egg yolks, cinnamon, ginger, salt, vanilla powder, pumpkin puree, $1/3$ cup maple syrup, and xylitol. Puree until smooth and pour about $2/3$ cup into each greased ramekin.

Place the roasting pan on a pulled-out oven rack and, with a pitcher or measuring cup, add enough hot tap water to reach halfway up the sides of the ramekins. Cover the pan loosely with foil punctured with several small holes and bake until the flan is set, 35 to 45 minutes. Let cool in the water bath for 20 minutes, then refrigerate for 2 hours.

Serve the flan cold in the ramekins with a drizzle of maple syrup.

SPICED BAKED APPLES

SERVES 2

Looking for a great applesauce? Just blend the baked apples and baking juices in a food processor until smooth. Be sure your apples are organic to minimize pesticide exposure.

1½ tablespoons ghee, melted

1 teaspoon Bulletproof Brain Octane oil (or MCT or coconut oil)

¼ teaspoon lab-tested, mold-free vanilla powder, such as Bulletproof VanillaMax

2 teaspoons fresh lemon juice

1 cinnamon stick

1½ teaspoons finely minced fresh ginger

2 organic apples (Honeycrisp, Mutsu, or Crispin are good choices), peeled, cored, and quartered

Preheat the oven to 325°F.

In a large 9 x 13-inch baking pan, combine the melted ghee, Brain Octane oil, vanilla powder, lemon juice, cinnamon stick, and ginger. Stir to combine. Add the apples and toss to coat. Turn the apples flat-side down. Cover the pan with foil and bake, turning halfway, until tender when pierced with a knife, 35 to 40 minutes.

Serve warm.

BULLETPROOF BLUEBERRY GELATO

SERVES 2 TO 4

What would July 4th be without dessert? Blueberries are antioxidant power-houses, and the anthocyanins that give them their brilliant blue color also increase HDL (good cholesterol) and fight inflammation. This recipe uses coconut milk to keep things light and refreshing. Be sure you get organic blueberries—nonorganic ones are high in pesticide residue, particularly if they're grown in the U.S.

10	ounces blueberries
½	cup plus 2 tablespoons canned coconut milk, well shaken
3	tablespoons Bulletproof Brain Octane oil (or MCT or coconut oil)
2	large pastured egg yolks
	Pinch of vanilla powder
3	tablespoons xylitol
2	grams (2,000 mg) ascorbic acid (see Note), for tartness

In a blender, combine all the ingredients and blend until smooth.

Pour the mixture into an ice cube tray (silicone is best) and stick in the freezer for 3 hours (or use an ice cream maker, if you have one).

Once frozen, put the cubes back in the blender and blend briefly, just until smooth.

NOTE: Ascorbic acid is vitamin C. If you take it as a supplement, you can just break open a couple of capsules.

SHOCKINGLY RICH CHOCOLATE TRUFFLE PUDDING

SERVES 4

When you use the best-quality ingredients, a dessert like this is a nutrient-rich food that will help you lose weight, instead of Kryptonite that will leave you inflamed and craving more. Tip: Use Bulletproof CollaGelatin to provide two times the protein of regular gelatin.

4	cups canned coconut milk, well shaken
	Up to 4 tablespoons hardwood xylitol or stevia (to taste)
1	tablespoon gelatin
2	teaspoons lab-tested, mold-free vanilla powder, such as Bulletproof VanillaMax
$^3\!/_4$	cup raw cacao powder, such as Bulletproof Upgraded Chocolate Powder
4	tablespoons grass-fed unsalted butter
1	tablespoon Bulletproof Brain Octane oil (or MCT or coconut oil)
$^1\!/_4$	cup macadamia nuts, plus more for topping (optional)

In a saucepan, combine 1 cup of the coconut milk, the xylitol, and gelatin and heat over medium heat until dissolved.

Pour the remaining 3 cups coconut milk into a blender and add the vanilla powder, cacao powder, butter, and oil. Blend thoroughly. Add the hot coconut milk/gelatin mixture to the blender and the macadamia nuts (if using). Pulse until mixed. Pour the entire mixture into a large bowl and refrigerate for 1 hour to set.

If desired, serve topped with chopped macadamias.

COCONUT-BLUEBERRY PANNA COTTA

SERVES 4 OR MORE

One of the best parts of the Bulletproof diet is being able to eat delectable desserts like this on a regular basis. Tip: Using grass-fed Bulletproof CollaGel-atin will provide twice the protein of normal gelatin.

1	cup fresh or frozen blueberries, plus more for serving
4	cups canned coconut milk, well shaken
	Up to 4 tablespoons hardwood xylitol or stevia (to taste)
2	tablespoons gelatin
2	teaspoons lab-tested, mold-free vanilla powder, such as Bulletproof VanillaMax
4	tablespoons grass-fed unsalted butter
1	tablespoon Bulletproof Brain Octane oil (or MCT or coconut oil)
$\frac{1}{2}$	cup unsweetened shredded coconut

Spread the blueberries on the bottom of a high-sided dish—an 8- or 9-inch round or square casserole works nicely.

In a saucepan, combine 1 cup of the coconut milk, the xylitol, and gelatin and heat over medium heat until dissolved.

Pour the remaining 3 cups coconut milk into a blender and add the vanilla powder, butter, and oil. Blend thoroughly and then add the hot coconut milk/gelatin mixture and the shredded coconut. Pulse the blender until mixed. Pour the entire blender contents over the blueberries and refrigerate for 1 hour to set.

Serve topped with more berries.

BULLETPROOF COLLAGELATIN BITES

SERVES 4 TO 6

Adding gelatin to meals adds necessary amino acids such as glycine, glutamic acid, proline, and alanine, which are often missing in the Western diet and which are essential to supporting the body's ability to repair and maintain healthy skin, joints, and bones.

- 3 cups of your favorite brewed mixed-herb tea (I love a blend of dandelion root, nettle leaf, ginger root, cinnamon bark, and fennel seeds)
- ¼ cup fresh lemon juice
- ¼ cup raw honey or hardwood xylitol
- 6 tablespoons Bulletproof CollaGelatin (or for less protein, 3 tablespoons generic gelatin)

In a saucepan, combine the tea, lemon juice, and honey and heat over medium heat until just warm, then reduce the heat to low.

Using an immersion blender, blend all the ingredients well until completely mixed. Add the CollaGelatin and mix until dissolved.

Pour the mixture into a pan or mold (an 8- or 9-inch round or square casserole works nicely). Let cool, then refrigerate for 2 hours to set.

Cut into bites and serve!

VARIATION

To make Lemony Hibiscus CollaGelatin Bites: For a relaxing afternoon or evening snack, replace the 3 cups of mixed-herb brewed tea and the lemon juice with 1 cup brewed chamomile tea, 2 cups brewed hibiscus tea, and ¼ cup fresh pineapple juice. Be sure to heat this mixture before refrigerating to deactivate the bromelain in the pineapple juice.

CHAPTER 10

SALTS, BUTTERS, AND CONDIMENTS

S pices and condiments often have medical or healing properties and part of the Bulletproof philosophy is to leverage these benefits and to avoid some spices that have more downside than upside. Feel free to figure out what works for you, but be aware of what the suspect spices like garlic and black pepper do—quality matters even more in those cases. That's why you won't find those suspect characters in here.

FENNEL SALT

MAKES ABOUT ⅓ CUP

I didn't grow up eating fennel seeds, but I came to appreciate them in Silicon Valley in Indian restaurants where they give you a handful after a meal. My kids love to eat them straight. Now I know the flavor does wonders for veggies. Also, the sumac here adds some pretty color.

- 1 tablespoon fennel seeds
- 1 tablespoon dried thyme
- 2 tablespoons plus 2 teaspoons coarse sea salt
- 4 teaspoons ground sumac (optional)

Combine everything in a spice grinder or in a small mortar. Pulse, or crush with a pestle, to a coarse sand. Store in an airtight container at room temperature for 3 weeks, or in the freezer for 2 months.

CILANTRO-LIME COMPOUND BUTTER

I tend to keep some of this in my freezer at all times. I love it that much. However, if you're one of the 20 percent who think cilantro tastes like soap, that's no problem. It's a genetic predisposition and this recipe simply isn't for you.

8	tablespoons (4 ounces) grass-fed butter, at room temperature
½	cup cilantro leaves, finely chopped
2	tablespoons grated lime zest
2 to 3	teaspoons fresh lime juice (to taste)
	Sea salt to taste
¼	teaspoon cayenne pepper (optional)

In a food processor, combine all the ingredients and pulse until well combined. Store in the fridge in an airtight container or wrapped in parchment for 5 days or in the freezer for up to 2 weeks.

BULLETPROOF CURRY POWDER

MAKES ABOUT ¼ CUP

There are probably 10,000 curry recipes around the world at this point, and they all center around these ingredients. Please don't take offense if this one differs from yours—it's not a traditional Thai or Indian blend. If you've never experimented with curry, this one uses the most Bulletproof spices. The only thing that might inspire more culinary passion for me than guacamole is curry. This one works every time.

1	tablespoon ground turmeric
1	tablespoon ground cumin
2	teaspoons ground ginger
1½	teaspoons ground coriander
½	teaspoon lab-tested, mold-free vanilla powder, such as Bulletproof VanillaMax
½	teaspoon sea salt (to taste)
¼ to ½	teaspoon ground cinnamon (to taste)
	Pinch to ⅛ teaspoon cayenne pepper (to taste), optional

Combine all the spices in an airtight jar, stirring or shaking well to combine. Store in an airtight container at room temperature for 3 weeks or in the freezer for 2 months.

SALSA VERDE

MAKES 1 SCANT CUP

This is one of the few salsa verde recipes that avoids tomatillos or any of its nightshade cousins. Capers taste great here and stay authentic to salsa verde tradition. If you know you're not sensitive to jalapeño and cayenne as suspect foods, feel free to spice it up.

1	scallion, sliced
$3/4$	cup fresh parsley leaves
$1/2$	cup fresh cilantro leaves
$1/3$	cup fresh basil leaves
2	tablespoons capers
1	tablespoon apple cider vinegar
5	tablespoons olive oil
1	tablespoon Bulletproof Brain Octane oil (or MCT or coconut oil)
	Sea salt

In a food processor, combine the scallion, parsley, cilantro, basil, capers, vinegar, and oils and puree to a coarse sauce. Season with salt to taste. Store the salsa verde in an airtight container in the refrigerator. Use within 2 days.

TAPENADE

MAKES ¾ CUP

I never understand why anyone would eat hummus when tapenade and guacamole are such better options. Tapenade adds great flavor and healthy fat to almost anything. Just be sure to use high-quality olives free of MSG.

1	cup pitted Niçoise or Kalamata olives
½	teaspoon fresh thyme leaves
2	teaspoons minced scallion greens
1	tablespoon Bulletproof Brain Octane oil (or MCT or coconut oil)
1	tablespoon high-quality olive oil
2	teaspoons capers

In a food processor, combine all the ingredients and pulse to a smooth, thick puree. Store in an airtight container for up to 1 week.

BULLETPROOF MAYONNAISE

MAKES ABOUT 1½ CUPS

If your mayo won't emulsify, try adding a chunk of avocado, an egg yolk, or some soy lecithin. I like to add fresh herbs to flavor my mayo, too! Unfortunately, this has too much protein for protein fast days.

1	large pastured egg
¾	cup extra light olive oil
¼	cup Bulletproof Brain Octane oil (or MCT or coconut oil)
2 to 3	teaspoons fresh lemon or lime juice
	Pinch of sea salt

In a bowl, combine all of the ingredients and let the egg sink to the bottom. Using an immersion blender, blend all of the ingredients until the mayo reaches the desired consistency. Store in the fridge.

IN CONCLUSION

I hope you're as excited about these recipes as I am. It's been a pleasure pulling them together for you based on years of playing in the kitchen. They are here not only for their amazing potential to help you hack your body, but also to be the most versatile, innovative, imaginative dishes they can be.

Dress them up, pack them up, share them, repurpose them, combine them, use them on fasts. However you like to live, eating a Bulletproof diet is easy and the dishes are adaptable to what you crave and what you love. Here's to hacking your way to your best self and loving every bite!

With gratitude, Dave

SAMPLE FASTING DAYS

BULLETPROOF PROTEIN FAST:
SAMPLE MEAL PLANS AND PROTOCOL

Here's a sample shopping list to stock up on in preparation for your big day of protein fasting:

Plenty of unsalted grass-fed butter

Sweet potatoes, yams, carrots, cucumbers, celery

Avocados

White rice (and fresh white rice mochi)

Low-fructose fruits: berries of all kinds, lime, and lemon

Bulletproof Coffee ingredients: Bulletproof Brain Octane oil, Bulletproof Coffee beans

The following sample meals will help your body detox even more efficiently while giving you an extra boost of energy.

1 BULLETPROOF PROTEIN FAST BREAKFAST

PROTOCOL: Choose one from below to have as soon as you get up or whenever you are accustomed to eating breakfast.

Bulletproof Coffee

Green tea blended with butter and Bulletproof Brain Octane oil (not as powerful as Bulletproof Coffee, however!)

2 BULLETPROOF PROTEIN FAST LUNCH

PROTOCOL: Choose one to be eaten 15 to 18 hours after the previous night's dinner.

Guacamole with cucumber and/or celery sticks

Sweet potato-ginger soup

Iceberg salad with baked carrot fries

3 BULLETPROOF PROTEIN FAST DINNER

PROTOCOL: Choose one to be eaten 5 to 6 hours after lunch.

Iceberg salad with buttered white rice

Carrot-fennel soup with white rice

Baked sweet potato with guacamole

4 BULLETPROOF PROTEIN FAST DESSERT (OPTIONAL)

PROTOCOL: To be eaten soon after dinner.

Bulletproof Berry Bowl: combine blueberries, raspberries, and strawberries with a squeeze of lemon juice and sprinkling of chopped fresh basil—enjoy!

HOW TO HACK YOUR PROTEIN FAST

Remember, your goal is to stay below 15 grams of protein total during your one protein fasting day each week. Some people find it hard to count to 15, or tell me they are too lazy to do so, so here are my favorite tips:

HACK #1:
Google It

If you want to eat something and you aren't sure if it has protein in it, I highly recommend the ancient biohack I like to call Google. You can simply type in "how much protein is in broccoli" or "protein in avocado"—or whatever you are trying to find out—to get an approximate measurement.

HACK #2:
Buy a Digital Kitchen Scale

By purchasing a small kitchen scale, you'll be able to measure out your portions of protein powders and other upgraded powders quickly and easily, which is useful for all Bulletproof recipes whether it's a protein fasting day or not.

HACK #3:
Re-Feed on Bulletproof Carbs Instead of Having a Junk Food Cheat Day

Keep in mind this is not a cheat day. Do not give yourself permission to hit up all of your local fast-food joints and then eat an entire cake! Bulletproof Protein Fasting is simply a great way to get an even better reduction in inflammation and superior Bulletproof results. Call it a cheat day if you want—but only in that not eating enough carbs will cheat your body out of what it needs to burn fat and rejuvenate its detox systems!

Like I always say: If you're hungry 2 hours after a meal, you aren't eating right. This guideline applies on all days of the week, even protein fasting day.

SAMPLE BULLETPROOF INTERMITTENT FASTING

Here is a sample day of Bulletproof Intermittent Fasting, which I explain in more detail below:

8 P.M.: Eat your last meal before beginning the fast the next day.

8 A.M.: Drink Bulletproof Coffee.

2 P.M.: Break the fast with Bulletproof foods.

Bulletproof Intermittent Fasting is the same as traditional intermittent fasting, except you consume a cup of Bulletproof Coffee in the morning. The healthy fats from grass-fed butter and Bulletproof Brain Octane oil give you a stable current of energy that sustains you through the day. The ultra low-toxin Upgraded Coffee beans optimize brain function and fat loss with high-octane caffeine. The Bulletproof Brain Octane oil also serves to increase ketone production and boosts your metabolic rate by up to 12 percent. This drink is so filling, we've had clients who drank one cup of Bulletproof Coffee in the morning and didn't feel like eating until midafternoon.

For optimal results, you should be follow-ing the green side of Bulletproof Diet roadmap (www.bulletproof.com/diet-roadmap-poster) in conjunction with this protocol. Bulletproof Fasting will not save you from the effects of Pop-Tarts and fried Oreos.

BULLETPROOF INTERMITTENT FASTING: MENTAL PERFORMANCE PROTOCOL

Goal: Improve and/or sustain mental performance while getting more benefits than from traditional intermittent fasting.

STEP 1: Finish dinner by 8 p.m. the night before

No snacking after dinner—go to bed whenever you want.

STEP 2: Drink Bulletproof Coffee in the morning

Bulletproof Coffee is a mix of brewed Upgraded Coffee beans, grass-fed butter, and Upgraded XCT oil (our pharmaceutical grade Brain Octane oil). You can find the complete recipe on page 166. Don't mess around with cheap coffee, which may sabotage your efforts due to mycotoxins.

Drink as much Bulletproof Coffee as you like in the morning. You can have another cup before 2 p.m. if you get hungry. But no coffee after 2 p.m. or you won't sleep.

STEP 2.5 (OPTIONAL): Work out

This is not necessary to gain muscle and lose fat, but it helps. If you're going to work out, I'd suggest high-intensity weight training right before you break the fast in step 3. Shorter and harder is better than longer exercise. You will need to sleep more if you exercise.

STEP 3: Eat lunch after 2 p.m.

This means you've not had anything to eat except Bulletproof Coffee for 18 hours. This should occur from the time you wake, through the morning, and into the afternoon. If 18 hours is too long, start with a shorter fast and increase from there.

STEP 4: Eat as much Bulletproof food as you like for 6 hours (until 8 p.m.)

The number of meals you eat during this time is irrelevant, as is the amount of calories.

ACKNOWLEDGMENTS

When you cook a Bulletproof meal for a person you care about, it's an act of service. You're doing one small thing just right that can help your friend experience a "food high" followed by amazing energy for an entire day, free from cravings and crashes.

When your friends experience a day like this, it makes them treat other people better too. Which makes those other people feel good, so they in turn treat other people better. This stuff matters.

All it takes is a meal that unlocks your biology so you have the energy and control you were meant to have. That's why I decided to create *Bulletproof: The Cookbook*.

Also, I wrote this because you can cook quality meats, fats, and vegetables simply and deliciously when following the Bulletproof Diet, but sometimes even grass-fed steak and broccoli just get old—and it's amazing to craft more delicious, creative options when you have the time to spice it up.

Special thanks to Brandon Routh, friend and Hollywood superhero. Brandon took time out of his busy filming schedule for his role as The Atom in DC's *Legends of Tomorrow* show in order to share his Bulletproof story, which you'll read about here. I was touched to hear how this work helped him and humbled that he was so willing to share.

Thank you to the entire publishing team who helped transform the idea for this cookbook into a reality. It was truly a group effort far more complex than even the most amazing French meal. Thank you to my beyond-fantastic agent, Celeste Fine; it is truly an honor to work with you every day, and I'm so glad J.J. Virgin introduced us. Thank you to the amazing team at

Rodale, led by Marisa Vigilante and Jennifer Levesque, for your hard work on this fantastic second collaboration together. Gratitude to Jamie Shaw, Ellen Scordato, and their entire crew for helping test and tweak these recipes to make them as perfect as they could be!

One enormous thank you to the entire Bulletproof team for making the cookbook launch such a success. A big thank you to Carrie Simons, Ashley Sandberg, and their wonderful team at Triple7 PR for getting the word out about all these delicious recipes and the way they upgrade human performance. Russell Brunson, I am grateful for your invaluable advice in the months leading up to the book launch—the entire Bulletproof team learned so much from your wisdom and strategic support.

To Zak Garcia, Nikki de Goey, Susan Lyon, Yo Fujikawa, Peter Bauman, Kailey Stein, Meghan Kelly, and every member of the Bulletproof staff who were instrumental in pulling off our second major book publication: You all helped make this happen and I am infinitely grateful! Let's all have a potluck at Bulletproof Labs to celebrate. I'll bring the guac! ;-)

Last but not least—and perhaps most influential in the recipe creation process—thank you so much to my wife, Lana, and kids, Anna and Alan, for being the best test kitchen and taste testers I could have ever asked for. ;-) They patiently put up with several "rough drafts" of each recipe before we finally perfected each one....

Thank you so much to all the wonderful people who came together to support this cookbook. Enjoy the feast!

INDEX

Underscored page references indicate sidebars. An asterisk (*) indicates that photographs appear in the color insert pages.

C

Cabbage
  Bok Choy Anise Soup, 156
  Braised Cabbage, 121
  Carrot and Cabbage Slaw,* 122
  Trout with Cabbage and
      Bacon,* 86
Cacao
  Bulletproof Coconut Hot
      Chocolate,* 168
  Shockingly Rich Chocolate
      Truffle Pudding, 195
Canola oil, 20
Capers
  Salsa Verde,* 203
Carbohydrates
  created from proteins, 4–5
  during protein fasting, 13, 13,
      211
  starchy, recommended servings
      of, 16
Carbohydrate vs. fat burning, 4
Cardiovascular disease, fats and,
      20
Carrots
  Carrot and Cabbage Slaw,* 122
  Carrot and Ginger Smoothie
      Soup,* 149
  Carrot and Sweet Potato Mash,
      127
  Coconut-Braised Mackerel and
      Quick-Pickled Carrots,
      106–7
  cooked, for smoothies, 164–65
  Winter Vegetable Salad,* 70
Casein, in dairy foods, 29
Cashew milk, 30
Cashews
  Cauliflower and Cashew Soup,
      151
  Rice Soup with Bok Choy and
      Cashews, 150
Cauliflower
  Cauliflower and Cashew Soup,
      151
  Cauliflower-Bacon Mash, 142
  Cauliflower "Couscous,"* 54, 117
  Curried Cauliflower Steak,* 113
  Trout Not-Fried Not-Rice, 87

Cayenne, 36, 52
Celery
  Simple Green Bulletproof Soup,
      154
  Sole with Celery Puree and
      Green Beans,* 83
Celery root
  Rutabaga and Celery Root
      Puree,* 116
Ceviche
  Bulletproof Ceviche, 100
Charred food, as carcinogenic, 42
Cheating, 17, 211
Chestnuts
  Chestnut Dumplings with
      Arugula and Squash, 108
Chicken
  Bulletproof Chicken, 104–5
  problems with, 27–28, 51
Chickpeas
  Warm Lamb and Chickpea
      Salad, 101
Chile peppers, 36
Chili
  Beef Chili, 90
  Braised No-Chile Lamb Chili,
      89
Chocolate
  Bulletproof Coconut Hot
      Chocolate,* 168
  Chocolate-Coconut Truffles,
      188
  Chocolate-Dipped Pears,* 189
  Chocolate-Drizzled Pear Salad
      with Lemon-Rosemary
      Vinaigrette, 140–41
  Shockingly Rich Chocolate
      Truffle Pudding, 195
  as snack, 20
  Vegan Chocolate Mousse, 190
Chowder
  Vietnamese-Style Fish Chowder,
      160
Cilantro
  Bok Choy with Cilantro-Lime
      Butter, 118
  Cilantro-Lime Compound
      Butter,* 55, 201
  Pork Belly Cilantro Stew, 94
  Salsa Verde,* 203

Cinnamon, 36, 38
Citrus, how to segment, 85
CLA, 23
Clafoutis
  Raspberry Clafoutis, 186
Cleaning products, toxins in, 45
Cloves, 38
Coconut
  Coconut-Blueberry Panna
      Cotta, 196
Coconut cream
  Berries and Coconut Cream,*
      181
  Chocolate-Coconut Truffles,
      188
Coconut flakes
  Coconut Smoothie,* 172
  Pork Flank Steak with Coconut
      Relish, 91
Coconut milk
  Bulletproof Coconut Hot
      Chocolate,* 168
  Coconut-Blueberry Panna
      Cotta, 196
  Coconut-Braised Mackerel and
      Quick-Pickled Carrots,
      106–7
  Coconut-Cranberry Soup,* 155
  Coconut Creamed Spinach,*
      114
  Coconut Crepes with Citrus
      Salad, 191
  Coconut Smoothie,* 172
  Turnip Gratin, 138
Coconut oil, x, 12, 16, 17, 20, 21,
      22, 24, 26, 51, 165
Cod
  Hake or Cod in Parchment with
      Salsa Verde, 81
  Wild Cod, Tapenade, and
      Butter-Poached
      Asparagus, 82
Coffee. See Bulletproof Coffee
Coffee drinks, flavored, 164
Coffee pot, for cooking eggs, 47
CollaGelatin
  Bulletproof CollaGelatin Bites,
      197
  Hibiscus CollaGelatin Bites,
      197

Food toxins, 6, 7. *See also* Mold
Fragrances, artificial, 45–46
Free radicals, 25, 36, 38, 39
Fruits, 30. *See also specific fruits*
    best to worst, 31
    Bulletproof Fruit Salad, 182
    limiting, 17
    organic, 15, 17
    recommended servings of, 16
    seasonal, for desserts, 177

G

Gelato
    Bulletproof Blueberry Gelato,
        194
Gentle baking, 42, 44
Ghee, 16, 17, 21, 23, 51
Ginger
    Asparagus in Ginger Broth,
        132
    Braised Lamb with Saffron and
        Ginger, 96
    Carrot and Ginger Smoothie
        Soup,* 149
    Ginger-Braised Ribs,* 92
    medicinal properties of, 37
    Romaine Salad and Ginger
        Dressing, 67
    storing, 37
    for sushi, 37–38
Ginger compress, 38
Gluten, xi, xii, 16
GMO foods, 20, 25, 28–29, 30, 40
Googling protein content of foods,
    211
Grain-derived oils, removing, 16
Grains
    best to worst, 33
    best types of, 31, 33
    fed to cows, 20, 22–23
    problems with, 30–31
Granita
    Pineapple Granita, 187
Green beans
    Chilled Poached Salmon,
        Watercress Sauce, and
        Green Beans, 79
    Sole with Celery Puree and
        Green Beans,* 83

Green tea
    Green Tea Latte,* 169
Grilling foods, 53
Guacamole, 20, 30
    Guacamole Crudités,* 63
Gut health, 35

H

Haddock
    Vietnamese-Style Fish Chowder,
        160
Hake
    Hake and Salmon Cakes,* 80
    Hake or Cod in Parchment with
        Salsa Verde, 81
Heart disease, fats and, 20, 25
Herbs. *See also specific herbs*
    Asparagus with Soft-Boiled Eggs
        and Herb Vinaigrette, 62
    for flavoring food, 17, 35
    Hanger Steak and Herb Butter,*
        93
    with medicinal properties,
        35–36, 38–39
    Pork Chops with Herb Crust and
        Wilted Dandelion Greens,*
        95
    raw vs. cooked, 35
High-fructose corn syrup, 40
High protein, high-fat diets, 6
Honey
    as dessert sweetener, 176–77
    for hacking sleep, 40, 176, 177
    Low-Carb Rice with Honey, 143
    raw, 40
Hot chocolate
    Bulletproof Coconut Hot
        Chocolate,* 168
Hotel hacks, 47–48
Hunger suppression, from
        Bulletproof Intermittent
        Fasting, 11, 13, 214

I

Ice cream
    Bulletproof "Get Some" Ice
        Cream, 180

Immersion blender, 164
Inflammation
    causes of, 8, 9, 26
    effects of, 35
    fasting decreasing, 11, 13, 14,
        211
    foods treating, 35
Inflammatory foods, in Bulletproof
        Roadmap, 15
Intermittent Fasting, Bulletproof,
        9, 10, 11–12, 213–14
Iron, for reheating leftovers, 47–48

K

Kale
    antinutrients in, 6–7
    Buttered Kale,* 125
    cooked, for smoothies, 164
    Kale Carbonara, 136
    Warm Steamed Kale and
        Pineapple Smoothie,* 171
Ketogenic diets, 4
Ketosis
    cycling in and out of, 4–5
    safety of, 4–5
    side effects of, 5
    XCT oil and, 12
Kid-friendly Bulletproof foods,
        55–56
Kitchen detox, 45–47
Kitchen equipment, 43–45
Krill oil, 17, 23–24

L

Lamb
    Braised Lamb with Saffron and
        Ginger, 96
    Braised No-Chile Lamb Chili,
        89
    grass-fed and grass-finished,
        28
    Lamb Cumin Loaf, 74
    Lamb with Cumin and Sumac,*
        97
    Warm Lamb and Chickpea
        Salad, 101
Lard, commercial, avoiding, 26